LOVE, SWEAT, AND TEARS

LOVE, SWEAT, AND TEARS

*How One OB/GYN Came Full Circle
in Her Love and Care of Women*

Pamela Dee Gaudry, MD, FACOG, NCMP
"America's Menopause Romance Doctor"

Savannah, Georgia
2017

Published in the United States of America by
Pamela Dee Gaudry, MD, FACOG, NCMP
15 Lake Street
Suite 160
Savannah, Georgia 31411

Library of Congress Control Number: 2015919694

ISBN 978-0-9970450-2-4 (Hardcover)
ISBN 978-0-9970450-3-1 (Softcover)
ISBN 978-0-9970450-1-7 (eBook)

Dedicated To

Allie

After listening to my stories for years, you were the inspiration for me to write for myself and, especially, to write for the women. For you, the name of this book will always remain, PAPS.

Robin, Quinetre, and Sarah

For laughing and crying with me and for helping me decide which stories were PAP worthy. Thank you.

Bonnie

For always being there. There are just no words. Thanks for the salt.

Mom and Dad

For being my biggest fans and never letting me entertain the thought that I couldn't do something.

Jonathan and Savanna

Of all the accolades that I have received in this life, nothing compares to just being your mother. I love you both so much.

Dana

For bringing unimaginable love, laughter, happiness, and joy into my life.

God the Father, Son, and Holy Spirit

For always being there through the triumphs and tribulations of my life, for giving me my family, and for giving me an opportunity to save some women. Thanks for the shove.

and

My Patients

For the love, trust, friendship, laughter, tears, and years. Thanks for the stories.

Endorsements

"Love, Sweat, Tears takes you on the exciting and truly heartfelt journey of a day in the life of a dedicated and beloved obstetrician/gynecologist, "Dr. Pam." You will be glued to your favorite seat as you get lost in this wonderfully told and incredibly educational piece; a must-read for all women."

Alyssa Dweck, MS, MD, FACOG
Gynecologist/Gynecologic Surgeon/Female Sexual Health
Assistant Clinical Professor Mount Sinai School of Medicine, New York
Massachusetts General Hospital Consultant
(Vincent's Memorial Ob/Gyn Service)

"Dr. Pam has written an amazing book! Yes, it's a great book on menopause; but it's also a great book on women's health in general, including sexual health and relationships.

It is also a wonderful book about what it is like being a female OBGYN. Our lives and our approaches to medicine are a bit different from those of our male counterparts—and Pam tells it like it is!

I also must say that I have always loved visiting in the South. When asked to speak with a group of women, or health care practitioners, I always am delighted when it involves a southern swing. Well, Dr. Pam's book exemplifies why I love visiting in the South: she tells it like it is, but in a very entertaining manner—and she makes it very clear! (And, there's always a wonderful accompanying story!)

So read this book! Just about everyone, female or male, will learn a lot about living a more enjoyable life."

Mary Jane Minkin, MD, FACOG, NCMP
Obstetrician/Gynecologist
Clinical Professor, Department of Obstetrics,
Gynecology and Reproductive Sciences
Yale Medical School

Love, Sweat and Tears *brings the art back to medicine . . . it's easy to begin thinking of physicians as disconnected and uncaring but Dr. Pam's book helps the reader believe again in physicians who want to build a relationship, share their passion and reassure you that no matter what you feel they will work with you to address the problem and help heal you.*

Dr. Pam is that physician and her story will leave you in tears of laughter as well as gratitude. Your "well-woman" checks will never be the same!!!

Mary Jo Rapini
Relationship and Sex psychotherapist
Author and Media expert

"*I have met quite a few doctors through the years, not too many gynecologists for obvious reasons, but countless physicians. I must say Dr. Pam stands alone with a unique approach to a woman's . . . Uh Hum . . . vagina. There I said it! And thank you Dr. Pam for your free spirit, funny take & brave story telling. To straight men out there— read this book!*"

Craig Shoemaker
Comedian
Author

"*This is the best book that I ever read!*"

Barbara
Dr. Pam's mom
Alert: Extremely Biased Evaluation

CONTENTS

FOREWORD

It all started with a cold call out of the blue. I heard a very pleasant voice accented with southern charm on the other end of the phone. She was asking about an interview for an upcoming film on menopause and sexuality. I knew from the first few moments of our conversation that this was not to be the regular interview. I thought our phone call was to last only a few moments, but about an hour later we were still chatting; we had become instant friends. Medicine and our mutual dedication for menopausal health and sexual wellness had made us colleagues, but Pam's kind and gentle personality coupled with her caring concern had made us fast friends.

I was fortunate to meet Pam in person for one of her first interviews for her upcoming movie, *Love, Sweat, and Tears*. She was travelling to Southern California and asked if I had the time to squeeze her in for an "in-person" interview. We scheduled a brief fifteen minutes for our conversation at the end of the day. Our interview lasted several hours as we shared laughter, personal stories of love, and friendship. It was as if we had been friends for a lifetime. This is how Pam operates both personally and professionally. This is how her book will captivate, entertain, educate, and nurture your mind, body, and soul.

I have had the pleasure of watching Pam during her journey from gynecologist and filmmaker to menopausal sexual medicine gynecologist. Her journey of academic and professional excellence was a marvelous story that unfolded with grace, charm, and panache.

Pam has a unique sense of medical commitment and dedication to duty that is rarely seen. She is a leader not only in her medical community, but somehow found the time to be on a local school board and volunteer as a den mother and Brownie troop leader. Everyone with whom she interacts is deeply touched. Pam is a hands-on clinician; she is a "hugger" of her patients! Anyone whose life she touches is forever changed influenced by her kinetic energy and style.

It is an honor and pleasure to have been chosen to write the foreword for her book: *Love Sweat and Tears*! It is a must-read for the menopausal woman as she lives life to its fullest in what Pam would call her "Jungle Sex Years!" Pam breathes life, humor, and medical accuracy into a topic that many women dread: Menopause! With humor, grace, style, and the unique gift of "honey bear" professionalism she will accompany you and your partner safely on your journey through the menopausal transition.

If a book would ever have the ability to reach out and hug the reader, make the reader feel connected with others, and give them that warm fuzzy feeling, this is it. This book accomplishes that special feat!

Sit back and curl up with a cup of coffee, southern sweet tea, a mimosa, or a nice Chardonnay and relax. Even if you are not a "hugger," this book and Pam will undoubtedly convert you. Prepare to be hugged.

Enjoy!

Michael L Krychman, MD, FACOG, NCMP
Sexual Medicine Gynecologist
AASECT Certified Sexual Counselor
Southern California Center for Sexual Health and Survivorship Medicine
Newport Beach, California

PREFACE

Why OB/GYN?

I knew that I was going to be a doctor. My first memory of wanting to do this was when I was eight years old. The little boy across the street from us, Michael, cut his leg open. All the kids in the neighborhood were at a house with a pool, and Michael came limping up with his leg bleeding pretty badly. I cannot quite remember how he cut his leg, but anyway, I ran up to him and brought him to the pool edge. I held pressure on the wound and used the pool water to clean off his leg. In my mind's eye I can still see the deep gash in his thigh. The color and texture of the tissue under the skin was mesmerizing, and I started pulling apart the wound a little bit to see what was under the first layer. I never noticed all the other kids in the neighborhood forming a semicircle around us and being totally grossed out by what I was doing. Someone said something like, "What are you trying to do, be a doctor?" and I was promptly pushed in the pool. What is wrong with that? I thought about it a lot after that event. I remember that I really wanted to see that tissue under the skin again.

During my sophomore year of high school, somehow I got a "pinkeye-like" infection in my eyes, and to my horror, my external genitalia also became infected. I could not go to school for about two weeks or so, and I was taken to several eye doctors and a gynecologist. I can remember being examined by ophthalmologists in the old hospital in downtown Savannah. Several gynecologists came to see me as well, and they talked to my mother as if I was not even there. No one could figure out what it could be, and I remember being very worried. The infection went away, and the doctors were just glad that it was "self-limited."

My brother and I went to the Bull Street Public Library after school. We would do our homework for a while and then my mom would pick us up. I loved the library. Besides getting my homework done, I loved the smell of the books and reading about anything. I loved reading encyclopedias; I loved going from topic to topic reading about so many things. Again, in my mind's eye, I remember getting the idea of looking up whatever virus I had acquired. In about ten minutes (remember, this was all the Dewey Decimal System, no Google or Bing), I found a medical book that described the "Adenovirus." The text described the uncommon infection in the eyes and the genitals. It was itchy, painful, and usually lasted two to six weeks. This was my first "Godwink." I think a Godwink is one of those events in your life that is too coincidental to be a coincidence. I really felt that God was talking to me and telling me that I was smart and that I should be a doctor. I immediately remembered little Michael and me in the pool. I immediately thought about all the doctors that examined my eyes and my genitals and wondered if any of them thought to pick up a book and read. It was another "calling" to the medical profession.

My next "calling" or "Godwink " was a major shove. I was a senior in high school, and although I considered myself "smart," I found myself worrying terribly that I was pregnant. I made my own appointment with a gynecologist. Not the same one my mom used—no discreet phone calls. I went into the office thinking that I was being very responsible and very "adult." Thirty minutes later the doctor told me that I was pregnant. I was hysterical and screaming to the nurses in the office that I had ruined my chances of going to medical school. What? I was worried about going to medical school? Where had that come from? The nurse in the office held me for about two hours. I calmed down enough to drive home. Forget medical school. I just realized that I was going to be killed by my parents and kicked out of school in my senior year. I got a grip, got myself together, put on my big girl panties, the ones that I should have kept on in the first place. I then decided that I was going to be responsible and act like an adult. I was going to take care of this situation. I was not going to tell anyone what had happened. I was not going to be kicked out of high school, I was not going to be killed by my parents, and I was going to medical school. What? There's that medical school thing again.

I was going to get an abortion and not tell anyone. The only problem was that an abortion was one of the worst things that I felt that I could do. I was extremely religious at a very young age. I was brought up as a Catholic, and I harbor a hefty dose of Catholic guilt. I went to a Christian school, and Jesus was discussed in just about every class. I knew Jesus would be upset with me. I prayed and prayed and prayed for Him to help me. My guilt was overwhelming, and I even thought about killing myself. I was having extensive conversations with myself and Jesus about which would be a worse sin, killing my baby or killing myself. I went to the abortion appointment thinking that I would spend eternity in hell either way and that I could not figure out how to kill myself anyway. I had the most wonderful doctor at the clinic. In my mind they would be old, dirty, and not talk much, but this man held my hand. He talked to me at length about my decision and wanted me to tell my parents. I poured out my soul to him. He took me into the exam room and, as I braced myself for another painful exam, he gave me the gentlest exam that I had ever had. I got up on my elbows and said, "You were so gentle!" Amazingly, he said, "I don't think that you are pregnant." I did another pregnancy test, and it was negative.

As he and the nurse walked me out to my car with me crying tears of joy and thanking God, I told him that I wanted to be an OB/GYN and be gentle to my patients as he was to me. He loved the compliment. Sadly, I do not even remember his name. With tears of joy streaming down my face, I drove to the OB/GYN's office to tell them the good news. The nurse there was so kind to hold me for so long, and I wanted to thank her. They brought me back to an exam room, and I told the doctor that my pregnancy test was negative at the clinic. He said, "I know that, I was just trying to teach you a lesson." The nurse and I both gasped. I got up and walked over to him and said, "I am going to medical school; I am going to be an OB/GYN. And I am going to save the women of Savannah from you." This event gave me the utter determination to make it. In the same day, I had encountered the nicest physician that I had ever met and the cruelest physician in the world. In a way this cruel physician pushed me hard to do well in school. Every time that I thought that I could not do it, I would think about that man taking care of young girls in Savannah, and it would push me on. This "Godwink" was my kick in the pants to do well in school because I had to come back to Savannah to save other girls from going through what I did. It could not happen fast enough.

ACKNOWLEDGMENTS

Most of this book has been written from the knowledge filed in the vast storage system located in my head. Unfortunately, these files are not accessible in any order. Since I have entered the menopausal phase of my life, I cannot remember who gave me most of the information or from which books I gleaned the knowledge. Actually, I can hardly remember much of anything. To all the professors and teachers at the University of Georgia that I encountered from August 1981 until June 1985, thank you. I would also like to thank all of my professors and teachers from the Medical College of Georgia from 1989 until 1993. I'm sure that I did not always like you, and I probably am still a little pissed off at some of you who made me cry. I may have even referred to you in disrespectful ways. For that, I am sorry. And yes, you are right, it was worth it.

As a Fellow of the American College of Obstetricians and Gynecologists (which means that I am Board Certified and adhere to a professional code of conduct for OB/GYNs), I have tried to write this book citing evidence-based medicine. That means that it is up-to-date knowledge on topics based on scientific evidence. I have used knowledge that was derived from investigators doing good studies using good statistical analysis. I have not included information that has not been supported by scientific evidence. When it is "how I do things," I have tried to simply acknowledge it. There is a wonderful web-based company called UpToDate. This company has made it very easy for physicians to get the most current information in the world on a topic. It does not make medical textbooks of medicine obsolete; they will be needed to teach students the basis of medicine in each topic. Medical information has increased tremendously in the last thirty years. Physicians cannot keep up to date on every topic. UpToDate gets the experts to write the most up-to-date information on a particular topic and to update the information when it becomes available.

When a physician pulls up a topic on UpToDate, they are informed exactly when the topic was last updated. As new evidence becomes available, all topics are updated. They are also informed when the last peer-review process has been completed. When an article is peer reviewed, it means that it was sent to many experts in the field who review it and check for inaccuracies. Suggestions are made for changes to the articles. If appropriate, changes are incorporated. It will be obvious to the reader when I have used information from the UpToDate article. I have referenced the title of the paper, the authors, and the dates through which the information has been updated. Lots of work goes into getting accurate information for this service. I appreciate all of the physicians, investigators, and statisticians who help with these articles. You have made the practice of medicine easier for the rest of us. This service is available through Wolters Kluwer Health. For the reader, please note that just because I practice medicine differently from your physician, it does not mean that your physician is wrong. We do it differently, because we were taught differently. Completely unlike eighth grade mathematics, in medicine there are many ways to get to the right answer.

I would also like to acknowledge Jim Stone and Scott Jacobs, who were instrumental in helping with completion of the book. In 2007 they founded Tytan Creates, a brilliant, innovative team of creative thinkers who have raised the bar for other branding and advertising companies. You know that it was a Godwink that we met you. I treasure your friendship.

Pamela Dee Gaudry, MD, FACOG, NCMP

THE BEGINNING

1
DELIVERY

I went to the University of Georgia for four glorious years. It was the most fun that I have ever had in my life. Athens, Georgia, and the University of Georgia are the best places in America. The University of Georgia Bulldogs is the greatest college football team on the planet. I feel sorry for young people who have to attend a different university. Tell your children that if they study hard in high school, they too can attend the greatest university in the United States of America. I had a wonderful gynecologist in Athens. He was also very nice and was so gentle. I was excited to tell him during my last visit with him that I was going to medical school and was going to be an OB/GYN. He tried to talk me out of it. He said that he loved his job, but it was very exhausting. He told me that I should go back to business school and be a stockbroker. Ouch. Burst my bubble.

That was in 1985. During the last twenty-five years, I have thought about that advice many times. I especially thought about that advice when I was awake waiting for a baby at four o'clock in the morning. That year I entered the Medical College of Georgia and embarked on an adventure of a lifetime. It was not the most fun that I have ever had.

The first two years were a combination of boot camp and prison. Many times I took tests for which I had not even finished reading the required material. I did not think that my brain could hold that much information. Whenever I thought that I could not do it, I thought of going home to Savannah. My "event" would vividly pop into my mind and give me the determination to keep going. I knew that I was doing the right thing because every time I learned about anything that had to do with the reproductive system, I could not get enough information. I loved hearing about women's health and obstetrics. My favorite part of anatomy was learning about the pelvic anatomy. It could not happen fast enough.

One of the best days in a medical student's life is when, in your third year, you get out of the classroom and go to the hospital. You get to wear the coveted white coat into the hospital. Third-year "clerkships" are when you are assigned a specialty, and you are on a "team" with other medical students from your class, residents in that specialty, and an Attending Physician. The clerkships are usually four to twelve weeks in length, and the student is assigned actual "patients" to follow while they are in the hospital. As my OB/GYN rotation approached, I found myself so excited and yet terribly apprehensive. I wanted to do a good job. I wanted them to like me. I wanted to like the rotation. I was frightened that I would not like it. What if I had come this far only to discover that I didn't enjoy the profession? I wanted a terrible lifestyle: long days in the office, up all night for many nights a month, and the stress of surgical patients.

My first day was one of the most exciting of my life. I arrived at the hospital to meet the intern at 5 A.M. We worked for the two hours prior to official rounds with the Attending Physician. First, we did all the circumcisions. I helped clean them up and then held them for a minute. We then went around on "work rounds," which meant that we saw all the postpartum patients, examined them, wrote notes, checked their labs, and got them ready for discharge. I worked hard, but not as hard as the intern did. We finished and ran to Labor and Delivery for official rounds with the Attending Physician, the "Attending." Every patient was formally presented to the Attending, who asked the residents questions about the patient and about obstetrics. They were continuously quizzed, and I learned so much just by listening. We then went around with the Attending and saw each patient briefly. The Attending was so nice to the patients. He held some of the babies and laughed with the patients. I could see myself in that place one day. After rounds, we admitted several patients who were in early labor. I was so excited that I might see a baby delivered. I happened to be "on call" that first night. This meant that I would spend the night in Labor and Delivery with the intern and see the patients that were in labor on a regular basis. We went around to each patient. We examined them and wrote a note on their progress. I could not have slept if I had wanted to. There was so much to do at night. The patients in Labor and Delivery were evaluated every two hours. The postpartum patients were seen for evening rounds, and all night, attention was directed to their needs. We saw patients who felt that they were bleeding too much, those with fevers, and those that were anxious and overwhelmed. We went to see gynecology patients in the emergency room and admitted those that needed to come into the hospital. We took care of the patients on the Gynecology wing and the Gynecologic Oncology wing that were having problems. At about 3 A.M. we were out on the floor seeing a postpartum patient. The intern was called to Labor and Delivery, and we ran back to the nurse that called him. When we got there, three women were all ready to deliver at once. Back then, all the patients went to the delivery room, and we gowned and gloved in surgical attire just as if it were a surgery in the main OR. The Attending was in the operating room downstairs in the main OR with the chief resident. They were operating on a gynecology patient. That left the third-year resident, the intern, and me to deliver the three patients that were ready. I had never seen a baby born. The third-year resident decided quickly that the two most experienced nurses would go into the room with me and, if for some reason my patient delivered prior to one of them getting there, I would have the best nurses to help. I was assigned to a fifteen-year-old girl who was having her first baby. They all thought that they would have completed their deliveries before my patient delivered.

Well, that did not happen. I scrubbed, got my gown and gloves on, and the nurses helped me put the drapes on the patient so that she was covered in sterile linens. The other two residents went into the other delivery rooms telling me that they would be right there. I was shaking. The nurses really did not think anything would happen either because the first baby takes a while to push down the birth canal, especially for a tiny fifteen-year-old who had great epidural and really could not feel a thing. The patient looked at me and said, "I think that I need to push." Before I could even respond, the vagina opened up and I saw the baby's head. I yelled for the nurses who were talking on the other side of the room. They ran over and just told me to grab the baby's head, support the head, and hold the baby as it came out. She delivered that baby in about five seconds. I put the baby on the mom's tummy, and one of the nurses held the baby there while I clamped and cut the umbilical cord. The baby went to the warmer and the nurse helped me deliver the placenta and check her for tears. She had no tears and her bleeding was normal. We cleaned her up and brought her back to the labor room to her family. They took pictures of me holding the baby and thanked me for helping her. I hugged them all. It was another fifteen minutes before the third-year resident came out of her delivery. She looked at me and said, "Good job!" I looked at her, still shaking, and said, "You can get paid for this?" She looked at me knowing how emotional I was, smiled, and just nodded her head yes. "It is the best job in the world," she said.

2
THE OBSTETRICIAN

During my senior year in medical school, I had to do a three-month internal medicine rotation. I had a good time with the Attending, the residents, and medical students who were with me on the rotation, but my heart was not there. One particular day on rounds made me realize that I was meant to be an obstetrician/gynecologist. Internal medicine rounds are extremely time-consuming. The residents and medical students go around the hospital ward, see all the patients, and write all the notes. Then the medical students and residents go around with the chief resident and we do the same thing again, and the chief resident learns about all the patients. Then the whole team walks around with the Attending Physician. It takes hours.

Anyway, we were finally ready to go on rounds with the Attending Physician. This was a time when the patients and families were in the room. Usually the patients and their families listened very closely to this conversation because the Attending Physician was asking questions to the residents and medical students. We would discuss the patient's diagnosis, prognosis, and plans for discharge. Often the patients or their families would also ask questions of the Attending. This was completely appropriate and sometimes very interesting. We walked into one man's room. He was probably about thirty-five years of age. He had a problem with his leg. He was in a fair amount of pain, and I cannot remember why his leg was injured. The Attending Physician was discussing his leg and the plans for evaluation. The whole time that the Attending was talking, this young man went on and on about the fact that nobody was listening to him, that he was not getting the pain medicine that he had anticipated, and that he felt that we were not taking good care of him. He never stopped whining the whole time that the team was in his room. It was horrible.

The Attending was trying to answer some of his questions, but every time the Attending started to talk, this young man would talk over him and start whining again. It was extremely frustrating for everyone, including me. At one point, when the whining was at its peak, I moved up to the man's bed, and I said, "For goodness sake, stop whining, it's not like you're in labor!" Well, you could've heard a pin drop in that room. I think that some of the residents gasped. The Attending decided to leave the room, and we all fell in line behind him. I was scared at the time, and I was wondering if I could be kicked out of medical school for something like that. I did not think before I spoke to the patient. It was one of the most frustrating conversations that I have ever witnessed. We got into the hallway, then the Attending called me over to the side by myself. I was shaking and very scared and trying to form the words in my head to explain my behavior. The Attending said to me, "First, thank you very much for what you did back there. I would appreciate if you did not tell the other residents that I was happy that you did that. I wanted to strangle that man. Secondly, I would like to know the specialty that interests you." I informed him that I was sure I was going into obstetrics and gynecology. He said, "I think that is a very good choice for you. I get the feeling that maybe you should not take care of men." I told him that I thought women were awesome, and I could not believe how much strength and courage they had when they were having a baby, had surgery, or were sick. He smiled and asked if I could turn around and act as if I had gotten in trouble a little bit. I did. From that day forward, when he talked to me, he called me "the obstetrician." My fate was pretty much sealed from that day forward.

When I was home visiting my parents on a holiday, we went down to River Street in downtown Savannah. I was shopping in one of the beautiful, quaint, gift shops down by the river. I looked up at the ceiling. Hanging from it were large, beautifully colored, quilted butterflies. They were individual mobiles to hang in your house. I assumed they were meant to hang over an infant's crib. I noted to my mother that those were the most beautiful butterflies I had ever seen. I walked out of the shop, but felt compelled to go back in and buy the butterflies. It was the strongest feeling I had had in a long time. I was supposed to buy those butterflies. I told my mother that when I had my own office, I was going to hang this from the ceiling in each room. I spent $400 on a credit card that I could not pay off. I bought every one of those butterflies in that store. My mother was in shock. I told her that I had to do it. I did not know why.

3
RESIDENCY

I entered my obstetrics and gynecology residency at the Medical College of Georgia on July 1, 1989. It was one of the happiest days of my life. Sometimes you get what you ask for. I do not think I ever worked so hard in my life as I did for those four years in that residency. The reason that they call the residents "residents" is because you become a resident of the hospital. During those years you spend much more time at the hospital than at home. Most of your meals are at the hospital, you sleep at the hospital, you shower at the hospital, and everyone wears scrubs. We usually did a thirty-six-hour shift every seventy-two hours. As with other medical and surgical specialties, the residents knew that there were 168 hours in a week and that you had to plan very well if you were to get enough sleep. My deepest and longest lasting relationships were developed during those four years. You spend more time with your fellow residents than you do your family. To this day I have a special place in my heart for each one of them. At the end of each month the attending physicians in the department would take the residents out at a local restaurant or bar to have a party. From our first day in this department, we were told that if we did not deliver a hundred babies a month, we would have to buy the beer for the party. We worked like a dog to make sure that we made our quota. I do not think anybody but our professors ever had to buy the beer, but we got very good at delivering babies.

The first two years of my residency I devoted mainly to obstetrics. During the third and fourth years I developed my surgical skills. Those two years were spent mainly in the operating room taking care of gynecology and gynecologic oncology patients. I still took obstetric calls at night, and there were several rotations those two years when you just do obstetrics. When a medical student picks obstetrics and gynecology as a career, he or she falls in love with delivering the babies. You do not fall in love with doing Pap smears and pelvic exams. I really did not know what to expect when I entered the gynecology part of my residency, and I was a little bit apprehensive. At this point, going into the operating room was not as exciting as delivering a baby. I was completely wrong. The first time I got that scalpel in my hand was one of the most thrilling things that ever happened to me. I thought back to the little boy across the street and cleaning off his wound in the pool. I finally was going to see what was underneath the skin.

The larger surgeries, such as hysterectomies and bladder tacks were reserved for the chief residents. The third-year residents were assigned to do the minor surgeries, such as D&Cs, tubal ligations, and diagnostic laparoscopies. I can remember the first time that I did an abdominal hysterectomy. The Attending Physician and the chief resident were on each side of the patient. The third-year resident, and I, the intern, were standing farther down on the side of the patient. The chief resident would be the "surgeon" and the Attending was the "first assistant" while he taught us all the steps for the surgery. The third-year resident was considered the second assistant, and the intern, the third assistant.

I was the third assistant. That means that I got to watch. My chief resident, who was my idol, asked for the scalpel, and we all waited for her to make the first incision on the abdomen. While I was looking at the patient's abdomen, she handed the scalpel back to the scrub nurse and said, "I don't feel so well and I think I need to lie down." The Attending Physician said, "That will be fine."

I was flabbergasted. Back then, it was a complete sign of weakness to get sick. Sometimes when we were sick, a fellow resident would put in an IV drip, and we would walk around with an IV pole so we did not get dehydrated. You never called in sick as a resident; if you were lucky, you were sent home. Therefore, you can imagine that this was unheard of in a surgical case. Anyway, she broke scrub and left the room. The Attending looked at the third-year resident, and said, "I guess this is your case now." She said, "I am not feeling well either." She left.

I can't believe this was happening. The Attending looked at me and said, "I guess this is your case now." I could see behind his surgical mask that he was smiling. I moved up the table to the spot where my chief resident had been standing, and I smiled too. To my surprise, everyone was waiting for me to ask for the scalpel. I did. I said, "Scalpel."

I can remember that surgical case like it was yesterday. When I look back on my life, this is one of the memories that comes to the top. The surgery went very well, and he talked me through every step. After the case was finished and we had cleaned up the patient and put the bandages on, I walked out of the operating room and headed to the recovery room to do the paperwork. To my amazement, my chief resident and third-year resident were sitting there laughing and talking to the nurses. She saw me looking at her, stopped talking, and walked over to me. She asked me if I had a good time. I did not understand. I just looked up at her and said, "Are you feeling okay?" She said, "Pam, I wasn't sick. We all decided that you had earned the chance to do a hysterectomy this year." It was all I could do not to burst into tears. I decided right then that I was going to do that for one of my junior residents when I was a chief. To this day, it was one of the nicest gifts that I have ever received. I finished my residency on June 28, 1993. There is a banquet at the end of the residency to celebrate each of the chief resident's accomplishments. Each chief is roasted in front of the whole department, the nurses from the hospital, and our families. After that, the attending physicians and the residents talk about the last four years. It is a very emotional and memorable event. Each chief resident gets a rocking chair with a plaque on the back that has your name, the years that you were resident, and the program name. This is a time-honored tradition in medicine and if you ever get the chance to go into your physician's private office, you will probably see a captain's chair or a rocking chair in a place of honor.

4
SAVING THE WOMEN

After my residency was completed, I took a few weeks off before I started my first official job at Memorial Medical Center in Savannah, Georgia. I spent most of my time sitting on the beach at Tybee Island, looking at the ocean, and doing absolutely nothing. I did go down to Florida for about ten days and learned to sail. This was the last time that I had absolutely nothing to worry about in my life. I started my first official job as a physician on July 23, 1993. I had my own desk that I did not share with anyone else, my own memo pads with my name on it, my own prescription pad with my name on it, and my own business cards. I still have the first of each memo pad, prescription pad, and business card in my desk. I hung up my butterfly mobiles in each exam room. I saw five patients that day. I spent about an hour with each of them, and typed up my own note instead of dictating one. I had never had to dictate an office note before, and I was scared of getting my note all screwed up on the Dictaphone. After all the patients were completed that day, I just sat at my desk. It was only 2:30 in the afternoon. My senior partner walked into my office and asked what I was doing. I told him that I really did not know. I did not really have anything to do, and for the last eight years of my life, I had never finished my day this early. He laughed and told me to go home. He said, "This isn't going to last very long, so you better enjoy a couple of early days for the next week or two before they get your schedule booked."

I did leave early for a couple days, but I felt incredibly guilty about going home. I should have taken his advice, because within two weeks I was seeing twenty-five patients a day and running around like a chicken with its head cut off. What I realized in that first month of private practice was that I really did not understand how good I had it in my residency. I did work hard; however, ultimately, the Attending Physician was really in charge, and every two to three months, I moved to a different clinical rotation. Any of the worries, frustrations, and difficulties that I encountered in a clinical rotation would eventually end, and I would start fresh on a new clinical rotation. Now they were my worries, frustrations, and difficulties, and they would never end. It was all my responsibility now; I was the Attending Physician. When an OB/GYN starts a new practice, their patients tend to be young. They usually are in their late teens to early thirties and are thinking about starting a family. You do have some older patients who are looking for a new gynecologist, but the majority of what you do is geared toward preventing pregnancy in young women and helping the rest get pregnant. Within a year I was managing about 120 obstetrical patients at a time. It was one of the best times of my life. If I was in town, I would do everything in my power to deliver my own babies. I used to get very upset when I missed one of my deliveries. Actually, I would be heartbroken. During a patient's pregnancy, the obstetrician and the patient become very close. It was not lost on me that this couple let me into the most intimate part of their lives for this brief period of time. I was with them when their child came into the world. That is an honor that I never took lightly. Whenever I delivered a baby, I felt that God was in the room. I felt that protective angels were present. I always looked up to the ceiling when the baby came out, just acknowledging that He was there with us, and I knew that He was just as happy as the parents to see His new child born. Obstetrics has to be the happiest medical specialty. Patients were typically young, healthy, and excited to be in my office. Almost every room that I walked into, the patient was overwhelmed and excited to see me, and I was excited to see them. It is wonderful to leave for home and know that I have affected so many lives in a positive way.

Patients sometimes ask if it is annoying to me to have to leave the office to do deliveries. To be honest, that is the most fun part of an obstetrician's day. Sometimes when the monotony of the office, the problems with the office staff, and dealing with insurance companies become too much, you are blessed with a call to Labor and Delivery to deliver a baby. The obstetrician runs to Labor and Delivery to do the one thing that we fell in love with—bringing a new baby into the world. Now, coming back to the office, with everyone sitting there waiting for you, there is a new anxiety. However, the women who are waiting know that their time is coming, and that one day you will be running to Labor and Delivery to deliver their baby. Women are the best.

5
SADNESS AND HAPPINESS

Of course obstetrics can be profoundly sad as well. The loss of the baby during pregnancy is devastating to the parents, the family, and the obstetrician. Patients may think that we deal with miscarriages all the time, and therefore, get used to this pain. You would think that after twenty years of being an OB/GYN I would have found profound and comforting words to give to the parents. I have not. Usually I am at a loss for words just as they are, and find that just giving both of them a long hug is all I can do. A miscarriage in the first trimester (which is up to thirteen weeks) is always sad and difficult, especially if it is not their first one. A miscarriage in the second trimester is so much more difficult to endure. The parents usually have told all their family and friends that they are pregnant, and they usually know if it is a boy or a girl. The patient looks pregnant, and has started to buy maternity clothing. A pregnancy loss in the second trimester may be more likely to have chromosome abnormality; however, it does not make the pain any less. A miscarriage in the third trimester (a fetal death) or shortly after birth (a neonatal death) is unbearable. I have somehow lived through five fetal/neonatal deaths with my patients in the twenty years that I have been an OB/GYN. I remember each one of them. Once I had children of my own, the memory of those five losses became even more painful. Now, I was not just feeling the pain from a doctor's standpoint, but from a mother's standpoint; the pain is still intolerable. The fear of every obstetrician is a difficult vaginal delivery. I think all of us have had difficult cesarean sections; however, there is always the realization that you can keep cutting on the uterus and you can eventually get the baby out. A difficult vaginal delivery may be one where the baby is too large to come through the birth canal. Sometimes the shoulder becomes stuck up in the abdomen behind the pubic bone. In this situation, the baby cannot get out of the mom's body. This is referred to as a shoulder dystocia and is a terrifying experience for everyone in the delivery room. The mother and the father know that you are struggling very hard to remove the baby from the vagina. There is usually a lot of yelling going on in the delivery room, and part of our protocol is to find another obstetrician to help. I am sure that it is frightening beyond belief to hear your doctor call for another doctor's help. There are maneuvers that OB/GYNs use to loosen the baby's position. We turn the baby, release the shoulder, and completely deliver the rest of the body. Usually everything turns out okay. Occasionally the baby's shoulder is injured, and he or she has limited use of their arm. Very rarely, you cannot get the baby out in time and the baby dies. Thank you, dear Lord, that this never happened to me.

This tragedy is only second to a maternal death. Most OB/GYNs will go through their entire careers and never lose a mother. When we hear of this happening either in our hospital, our community, our state, or somewhere in the country, I am sure that all obstetricians stop, pause, and say a little prayer for the mother, the family, and the obstetrician involved in the case. These are usually unexpected problems such as a severe hypertensive disease of pregnancy called eclampsia, a pulmonary embolism, or an amniotic fluid embolism. These problems occur quickly and sometimes without warning. In most cases it does not matter if the patient is in a small, rural hospital or in a major tertiary medical center with the most experienced doctor in the country. When one of these problems occurs, there is not much that the physician can do to help her. In OB/GYN (and probably in other specialties) we have what physicians call a "second victim." It is the doctor. When there is a bad outcome for the baby or the mother, people do not realize that the obstetrician is severely affected.

There are many reported cases where the obstetrician involved in a bad outcome stopped obstetrics and/or the practice of medicine. Most women know that there is a serious bond formed between the patient and her obstetrician. The obstetrician feels the pain of a fetal, neonatal, or maternal death as much as any member of the family. In obstetrics this problem is so widespread that our national organization has developed a network of other obstetricians for these doctors to talk to about their experience. Many of my patients and their families have asked me about how difficult it is to pay for malpractice insurance or asked if I am angry about how much insurance I have to pay. I have always responded that I felt that liability insurance was part of the cost of doing our particular business. I do not practice medicine trying to prevent bad outcomes so that I am not sued. I practice medicine to the best of my ability. Fortunately ninety-nine percent of obstetrics is happy. I have the most wonderful memories of delivering babies and taking care of "my women." I have two large photo albums filled with baby pictures. On the back of most of these pictures are the names of the babies, the parents, and a little note of thanks. I cannot spend more than about ten minutes reading these notes without bursting into tears. They are wonderful tears of joy and thankfulness for these people, who, for about a year, allowed me to share the most exciting time of their lives. I still take care of many of these patients and have the honor of getting follow-up pictures every year. One of the nicest pictures that I received was in a graduation invitation. The girl that I delivered and her mother sent me her high school graduation announcement with her newborn picture next to her graduation picture. It still brings tears to my eyes. I am thankful for their thoughtfulness. One special delivery comes to mind. I had been taking care of this young girl since she was sixteen years old. Unlike many girls her age, she longed to be a wife and mother; she could not wait to have children. At about the age of eighteen, she entered into a long-term relationship. After several years of seeing her only once a year, I asked when they were going to get married. I had always remembered that she wanted children. I think her story stuck in my mind because most girls her age were doing everything they could to prevent having a baby for the next fifteen years. Having children was on her radar from a very young age. She did come in one year and tell me that she finally got married, after a ridiculously long eight-year engagement, and I was very happy for her. I told her to enjoy this part of her life with her husband, because everything would change once she started having children. She looked at me, and tears formed in her eyes. She informed me that three months after they had married he moved to Washington, D.C. without her. She was devastated.

Here was one of those times that I spoke before thinking. I was doing her pelvic exam at the time, and I reached out and pushed the sheet down between her legs so I could see her face. I looked her straight in the eye and said, "This should be the best time of your life, and you only live once. I am not sure this man really wanted to marry you after waiting so long after your engagement to get married. If I knew how badly you wanted children, then I am sure that he knew how badly you wanted to have children. To up and move to another state without you is telling me that he does not want to continue his life with you. He sure does not want to have children. You need to leave him, get back out there, and find somebody that has the same goals and values that you do. You are a beautiful and amazing woman that deserves an amazing man. He is obviously not amazing; he is nowhere near the caliber of person that you are. Over the years I have watched many girls fall in love, marry, and have children. No one has wanted to do that as much as you have. Something is very wrong with this relationship, and I think you should get out of it."

23

I gave her my cell phone number to call me if she wanted to talk. I held her while she cried and cried and cried. I hurt for her as if she was my own daughter. I thought about her throughout that long day. I got in bed and said a little prayer for her. To my surprise my phone rang. It was late at night, and I was not on call. Even more to my surprise, it was the patient that I had given this abrupt and spontaneous advice to earlier in the day. She was crying hard, but she managed to tell me that she had called her husband and left him. I felt terrible. It hit me quite hard at that moment that my words were important to people. Young girls saw me as a role model and mentor, and my advice was probably taken more seriously. I was "their doctor." My words that I had always used to help others could also be used to hurt. I thought about it after I hung up the phone. I had been talking to her as a friend. I saw her as another woman (albeit, much younger than me) who was being treated terribly, and my instinct was to give her my advice. She took that advice and acted on it. I felt bad about that for many long months. I ran into my patient and her friend at the beach later that summer. She burst into tears when she saw me, but she thanked me for giving her the advice. She knew that it was the right thing to do; she knew that what I told her was right. I cried as hard as she did and told her that I was sorry that I had given her the advice without thinking it through very much. I told her that I really was talking to her as a friend and not as her doctor. I wanted her to know that I learned something from that encounter and that I would be much more careful in the future with other patients. She went into the nearby bathroom to freshen up, and her friend told me that her friends and family had been telling her that he did not want children and did not want to be married for years. She told me not to feel so bad because her family and all of her friends knew that I was the straw that broke the camel's back. When even her doctor could tell that she was in a bad marriage, she knew that what her family and friends were saying was correct. I thanked her friend for sharing this with me; it gave me some peace. Fast forward approximately two years and visualize this patient walking into my office. She looked at me with an awesome, mischievous smile and said, "I met someone wonderful." She told me all about him during her visit, and I commented that I had never heard her talk about anyone in this fashion. Later that year I got the most beautiful card for Christmas. It was a letter from this patient and her new fiancé. They both wrote part of the letter. They thanked me for my guidance in the past, and let me know that they planned to get married and have children. I had the honor of attending their wedding. I was honored again by delivering their two children. It doesn't get better than that. Another patient, her husband, and I were together through the course of five miscarriages over several years. It was heart-wrenching. She finally became pregnant using a donor egg. Unfortunately, my husband was very ill during her pregnancy, and my partner had to take care of her. I got a call from my partner one morning, and she asked if I wanted to do something special. My patient was having a scheduled cesarean section later on in the day, and she wanted to know if I wanted to do the surgery with her. That was a beautiful delivery.

Their daughter is now four years old, and when my patient is due for her annual exam, she brings her husband and daughter with her. We schedule her for the last patient of the morning and, after her exam, the four of us have lunch together.

6
LAUGHTER

Obstetrics is funny! Things, however, are usually funny long after the fact. You cannot deal with that part of the body, talk about that part of the body, operate on that part of the body, and deliver babies from that part of the body without funny (and sometimes, unfortunate) things happening. I was doing a cesarean section one morning and everything went perfectly. I had gotten into a habit of pulling the baby out of the uterus and abdomen, quickly wiping the baby off, and then having the anesthetist pull down the drape separating the patient and me so that she could see her new baby right away. On this particular day I did just that. I pulled the baby out of the uterus and abdomen, wiped him off quickly, and promptly held up her new baby boy. Her new baby boy promptly urinated in a perfect arc into her mouth that she had opened in awe of seeing her new child. She is an artist and she drew a picture of the event.

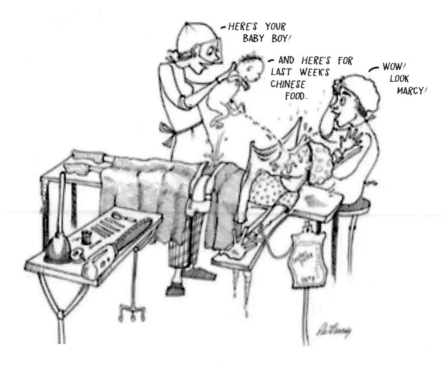

Another morning I was walking down the hospital corridor on the Labor and Delivery unit. I had a big day and I was making rounds very early in the morning. As far as I knew I was the only obstetrician on the unit. I said hello to many of the nurses. I went into my patients' rooms, examined them, and then went to the nurse's station to write my notes. On my way out of the unit I walked past a patient's room, and the nurse ran out into the hall screaming. She grabbed my arm, pulled me directly into the room, and pushed me between the patient's legs, which were up in stirrups. Without asking me, the nurse told the patient that it was okay to push now, and, with me fully clothed, the patient pushed hard. In one quick second, her water broke, and the baby came out quickly into my arms. I had amniotic fluid dripping through my hair and off my eyelashes. It went down my shirt, pooled in both of my bra cups, and then seeped down into my pants. My socks were wet. Every obstetrician has been in this situation; it is usually when you are in a hurry and have to be back to the office to see a full load of patients. You run to the call-room, take a shower, put on scrubs, and go.

Men can be very funny in the delivery room. I can remember on one occasion asking the father if he would like to come down between her legs and help me deliver the baby. When everything is going beautifully, I would frequently ask the father and mother if "Dad" would like to help me deliver the baby. If they are both okay with it, I would have the father put on a surgical gown, surgical gloves, and covers for their shoes. I would have him join me, in the quarterback stance. I would put his hands on the baby's head and guide the baby out. He would hold the baby for a second, everyone took pictures, and then I would lay the baby on the mother's belly and help him cut the cord. What could be better than delivering your own baby? The pictures were great, and I think that it was very special for many of the fathers. My biggest fear was the father passing out and dropping the baby so I would always have a grip on the baby's leg. Sometimes I was surprised by the fact that the father did not want to see the baby born. For example, when I asked one father if he would like to deliver his baby, he said, in a very concerned and profoundly caring voice, "Oh my God, I am not going to look down there. I worship that part of her body and I cannot bear to see it distorted in any way. Absolutely not." Wow. I don't think that anyone has ever worshipped a part of my body to that extent. I was impressed. Okay, stay up there and hold her hand.

One time I asked a father if he wanted to come down and help me deliver the baby, and he said, "I'm not looking down there until it has gone through a couple of car washes." He may never have sex again, with her. It is funny now.

Another father was watching me while I was sewing up a tear on her bottom after the baby was born. He looked a little queasy when he saw how open her vagina had become. He said, "It's not always going to look that way, is it?" I said, "I'll fix it up. You will not even know the baby came through here."

Yeah right. If you have had a baby, you know that it will never be the same. After those couple of these encounters, I was a little more cautious when encouraging them to look between the legs.

7
HE'S GOING DOWN

During the course of an obstetrical career, many men are going to faint in your office. Some faint when they see blood, some faint when you talk about "lady parts," and some faint when they see their wife having a pelvic exam. It is a little funny (after the fact) because they are usually coming there to be the strong protector for their wife. They are going to listen to the doctor, interpret what was said, and help make the decisions about the pregnancy. I am sure that it is humiliating to be in this position and then wake up on the floor with your legs elevated over your heart.

My best "man fainting in the office story" occurred while I was doing an amniocentesis. We were in a very small room. I was on one side of the patient and the nurse was on the other side holding the ultrasound wand. The ultrasound was used to find an area in the womb that was free and clear of baby parts and the umbilical cord. I then would put a long, thin needle into the womb and draw out a small amount of amniotic fluid. This was performed to make sure that the baby did not have any chromosome abnormalities. The patient's husband was in the room with us sitting on a chair. He asked if he could stand up next to her head so that he could comfort her and hold her hand. This was never a good idea because you could never trust a man not to faint during a procedure. It was against my better judgment. However, I let him do it because he told me the following story. "Doctor, I am a dentist, and dentists put those giant needles through your gums and into the nerves of your head when we are working on teeth. I am used to seeing large, long needles on a daily basis. This one going into her stomach is not going to bother me at all." Famous last words. The room was so small that in order for me to let him get up by her head, I had to walk out of the room and let him go past where I was. Then I reentered the room. He was leaning down talking softly to her and reassuring her that everything would be okay. The nurse and I resumed looking for an area in which to put the needle. We found the perfect spot, and I cleaned her belly over this spot with betadine and numbed up the skin with some local anesthetic. I then took out the needle, and under ultrasound guidance, pushed the needle through the skin of her belly, through the wall of the uterus, and into the amniotic cavity. Just when I was going to withdraw some fluid into the syringe, the crash occurred. He fell down on the side of the bed and rolled onto the floor. I knew that he was breathing because he was facedown and he was sucking the floor with each breath. I had the needle in her belly, so I could not stop and help him. I gently used my foot to turn his head to the side so that he was not sucking the floor. I finished withdrawing the amniotic fluid with some difficultly, because my patient was laughing hysterically. The more she laughed, the more me and the nurse laughed as well. We secured the amniotic fluid into the appropriate containers, moved the ultrasound machine so that we could get to him, turned him over onto his back, and placed the lower part of his legs on the chair that he originally was sitting on, the same chair that I should have kept him on for the procedure.

He woke up with me looking down at him. I had strategically placed my face above his face. As he opened his eyes, he looked directly into my eyes, and, hearing his wife laughing hysterically, quickly had full realization of what had happened. He said, "You aren't going to tell anybody about this are you?" I proceeded to tell him that I was going to tell everybody about it, but I would be sure not to use his real name. I told him that I would be sure to tell the part about him being a dentist and sticking those long needles through our gums and into the nerves of our heads. I hope he reads this and gets a chuckle, because I have thought about this procedure numerous times over the years and always get a good laugh.

8
EXPERIENCES OF A LIFETIME

Another time, I had just delivered a patient's baby. She had a small tear at the bottom of the vagina that I was meticulously sewing closed. Without any warning at all, she sat up in bed, looked at me, and vomited right on top of my head. She lay down while crying her eyes out, because she was terribly humiliated about throwing up on her doctor. The nurses got me a towel, and I cleaned up the best I could. I went to the call room, took a shower, put on scrubs, went back to her room, and finished sewing her up. I got a giant basket of beautiful, great smelling bathing supplies, fancy shampoo, and conditioner at her postpartum visit.

One of the greatest honors that an obstetrician can have is when a mother and father name their baby after you. I have had this profound honor on two occasions. I have kept in touch with those families. I have pictures in my office of me holding my namesakes. One of those patients had two boys that I had delivered. Although the child was a male, they used a variation of my name. During the course of her two pregnancies and deliveries, she had explained how much she wanted a girl. I came into her room the morning after her delivery, and she and her husband sat me down and told me that they were going to name their baby after me. I was overwhelmed. I cried. It was the best compliment that I have ever received. After I regained my composure, I talked to her about her tubal ligation that she had scheduled for that morning. I did not want to do the tubal ligation. She had wanted a girl so badly, but they felt that they could not afford another child. I thought that this was a bad time to make this decision. If they felt the same way in a year or two, we could do it then. They were committed to the sterilization. When it came time for her surgery, I accompanied the nurses to her room to transport her to the operating room. The whole way down the hall, I talked to her about this poor decision. She insisted that she wanted to have her tubal ligation. They took her to the operating room, placed an intravenous line, and prepared her for spinal anesthesia. I had been scrubbing my hands at the scrub sink with a heavy heart. The anesthesiologist does not put the spinal anesthesia into the patient until the surgeon is all scrubbed and ready. I came into the operating room holding my hands up in a sterile fashion. I calmly took the towel to dry my hands and arms. While I was doing this, I was talking to the patient about what a poor decision this was for her. She clearly became angry with me, pulled her intravenous line out of her arm, and walked out of the operating room naked with her arm dripping blood. Remember, this was about two hours after they sat me down and told me they were naming their child after me. She did not have the surgery. Eventually, she got over her anger, moved on, and I delivered her sweet baby girl about two years later. It doesn't get better than that.

Delivering a baby for a couple is one of the most rewarding experiences a physician can have; you become part of that family's lives forever. I understood that personally after my partner delivered my own children. I looked at him after the delivery, and I said, "I will never again refer to you as my partner, because for me, you will always be my doctor." I do not like to do tubal ligations. Sometimes, there is too much regret. I spent years talking one girl out of doing a sterilization procedure. In her defense, she did try everything else. She tried oral contraceptive pills, the contraceptive shot, and both a copper and progesterone IUD. I did put her off for about five years. She had never had any children, and I was worried that she would regret sterilization. She did her homework and came in with the following poster: 11 x 14 inches, complete on foam board and framed.

Top 10 Reasons to Feel Good about Permanent Tubal Sterilization for Anna
- Women > 30 years old are *less likely to regret* tubal sterilization.
- Women who make an *informed decision themselves* to have tubal sterilization are less likely to regret the decision.
- Anna has *never liked babies*—even the ones she's related to.
- Anna *will never have a baby* to make some future partner or her parents happy.
- The lower failure rate (compared to spring clips) could prevent *a termination of a pregnancy.*
- Anna is as stubborn as a mule and *refuses to use any form* of hormonal contraception.
- Anna is stubborn as a mule and *refuses to have any more foreign bodies* in or around her reproductive system.
- A signed and dated copy of this list can be added to *Anna's medical record* to document her extreme stubbornness regarding this procedure.
- Anna had this board professionally made because she is *so sure she never wants to be pregnant.*

I tied her tubes; it has been about five years now, and she is still happy. I stopped feeling bad about it. My reluctance to sterilize women does not have anything to do with my religious beliefs. I just changed my tune after the fifth woman and her husband came into my office (after her tubes were tied) and asked if I knew of any babies that they could adopt. That hurts. I devoted my life to bringing babies into the world. A progesterone IUD is a much better option. You get five years of birth control and very little menstrual bleeding.

9
THE GREATEST OBSTETRICIAN

One of my most favorite delivery stories (or really the one that affected me the most) involved a woman that was not even my patient. She and her husband were very young and very religious. They were both very adamant that she not have any medication during her labor and delivery. They had made a conscious decision that they did not want to expose their child to any drugs. Well, to the obstetrics staff and physicians, this is a routine story. We hear women come in all the time with birth plans mapping out exactly how they want their labor and delivery to go. The joke in labor and delivery is that the longer and more involved a woman's birth plan, the less likely that it will go how they would like it to go. Usually, as soon as the mom starts having real labor pain and starts screaming in pain, an epidural is not far behind. I have seen ten-page birth plans being ripped up by the patient and thrown at her husband. The poor husband usually is yelled and screamed at until the epidural is placed. With this particular couple, we all felt that it was going to be the same story. They were young, stubborn, and ill-informed. In this circumstance, when the mother is begging for an epidural and the father refuses, he does not look so good in the eyes of the Labor and Delivery staff. I am sure that they made a pact before they came to the hospital that even if she screamed she would not get an epidural, and it was his job to make sure that it did not happen. In this case it became apparent that she was in obvious pain, but she refused offers for pain medication and for epidural anesthesia. She became completely dilated (10 cm), but the baby was very high up in the pelvis. We had her start pushing, and the baby's heartbeat dropped from a normal of 120 to 160 beats per minute to a low of 70, then 60, then 50 beats per minute. Because I had just checked her cervix and told the nurse to start pushing with her, I was still in the labor room when the heartbeat dropped. There were two labor-and-delivery nurses, her husband, the anesthetist, the anesthesiologist, and myself in the room. One of the nurses appropriately called the neonatal intensive care unit and asked for their help immediately. We needed them to come to Labor and Delivery because, if we had to do an emergency cesarean section, we would need their expertise to take care of the baby. While she was on the phone with the neonatal intensive care unit, the other nurse and I started doing the usual things to get the baby's heartbeat back up. We rolled her on her left side, increased her intravenous fluids, stimulated the baby's head, and called for the staff to prepare for an emergency cesarean section. In this situation we usually place the patient on her bed and roll her back to the operating room, and if the baby's heartbeat has come back up, we will let her labor in there. However, if it does not come back up, we can proceed with an immediate cesarean section. In this case the patient was very lucky that the anesthesiologist had happened by to check on her and was readily available. To our surprise, both she and her husband calmly stated that they would not be going to the operating room. They had made a decision that, no matter what, they would deliver this baby vaginally. At this point, the baby's heart rate had dropped to forty beats per minute. That is too low. Oh my God, I can't take it. I calmly— I was not calm at all—tried to explain what a dire situation this was becoming. The baby was too high in her pelvis for me to put on forceps or a vacuum device to help her deliver the baby. They both calmly replied that they were thankful for my advice, but they were not going to take it. You could have heard a pin drop in that delivery room. One of the nurses started to cry. No one knew what to say or what to do. You cannot operate on a woman when she has refused. It is different if someone is in a car accident, and he or she is unconscious. In this case, the patient was fully awake, not sedated, and fully in charge of her own health care. (Inside, I was frantic.)

I know that I started to cry a little. As I was about to plead for her to listen to me, her husband turned to the window. He got down on his knees, folded his hands, looked up, and prayed. He said, "Dear Jesus, we really need your help right now. The baby needs to come out right now because the heartbeat is very low. We do not want our baby to die unless that is your will. You know that we were very anxious about getting our baby any medications, and we still do not want to do this. The doctor has advised us to prepare for a cesarean section, and we do not want this to happen. Could you please come here right now and help our baby come into the world so that we can start our family."

The baby moved in the abdomen and started down into the pelvis. With one push, she pushed that baby into my arms. She and her husband were both praying aloud when this happened. It was very good that the baby was crying very loudly (reassuring me that he was okay), because I was crying too hard to clamp and cut the umbilical cord. I asked for the nurse's help, and between the three of us crying with unbelievable emotion, we got the cord clamped and cut and handed the baby to the neonatal nurses who were still in attendance. There was not a dry eye in the room. The father got down on his knees again, and this time so did everyone else. He said the most beautiful prayer of thanks that I have ever heard in my life. I always believed that Jesus was in the delivery room when a baby was born. In this delivery, Jesus delivered the baby Himself.

10
PICTURES AND BUDWEISER

One of the best parts of the obstetrical care is the postpartum visit (the visit at six weeks after the delivery). It is so much fun to see the patient again. It is an "obstetrical law" that she must bring the baby for everyone in the office to hold and fuss over. She usually brings her picture album showing the pictures from the delivery, we take a picture of me with the baby, and I get the coveted newborn picture. It is a bit upsetting for an obstetrician not to get the newborn picture. We like to add it to our bulletin boards in the hallways for everyone to see. I compare the newborn picture to the football players stars, or stickers on their helmets in college football. For instance, when a University of Georgia Bulldog player is responsible for a major play, he gets a bone-shaped sticker for his helmet. It makes all the fans feel good about their team if their players have many stars, or bones, if you are a Georgia Bulldog fan, on their helmets. I think the patients feel good about their doctor when they see many healthy newborn pictures on the wall. As a thank-you, many families like to bring a small gift to their postpartum visit. The patients usually called my nurse to ask what kind of wine I liked to drink. They were always surprised to find out that, although I like wine, it usually makes me sneeze. I prefer to drink beer, specifically, the king, Budweiser. During the years that I was actively delivering babies, the word got out, and I always had lots of Budweiser to drink. Most of the mothers and fathers were embarrassed to give me the gift. My beautifully wrapped-up six-pack of Budweiser was usually handed to me with the words: "I can't believe I'm giving my doctor a six-pack of beer. We had planned on giving you a fine bottle of wine for you and your husband." I always reassured them that they had given the perfect gift. It was just a little difficult, however, to explain to new patients who came into my private office after their first exam why there were usually four or five six-packs of Budweiser next to my desk. My patients have been taking care of me over the years as well. I can vividly remember when I got married how happy they were for me, and when I got pregnant with twins they cared and worried about me as if I were part of the family. My two children have some of the most beautiful handmade quilts and blankets in the world. I actually have two hope chests filled with these precious gifts. I plan to give these back to them when they are having children of their own. When my husband became sick with cancer, my patients came to my rescue. They were always bringing food to the office and sending cards in the mail to help my family. When he died six years later, I had the most wonderful support from my patients. They felt that they were repaying me for what I had done for them. I wish that I could thank each one of them in person for their support. My patients have given me the most wonderful life that any doctor could have. It is an honorable profession.

11
GYNECOLOGY

Up to this point I have really left out the practice of gynecology. When you have a busy obstetrical practice, the gynecology part becomes secondary. I hate to admit that.

An OB/GYN tends to grow older with his or her practice. It is not that the gynecology patients are not as important as the obstetrical patients; it is just that obstetrics takes up most of your time, causes you to run from place to place, and makes you worry. There are probably OB/GYNs out there who have a busy gynecology practice from the beginning, but I suspect most of us start out doing 90 percent obstetrics, and when we retire, we are doing 90 percent gynecology. When patients come back for annual exams, and you have previously delivered their children, it is wonderful to catch up with pictures and stories from their children's lives. This is a very big part of the annual exam for an OB/GYN. As I have said previously, you become part of that family's lives. An OB/GYN is included in many of the milestones that a child reaches. I have gotten announcements when a baby has walked, when they entered kindergarten, when they graduated from kindergarten, and when they entered high school. I have received little notes in the mail when a child made the honor roll, when they became the quarterback for the high school football team, or if they had dance recitals. I have been invited to numerous high school graduations, college graduations, and marriages. I have been notified when a child that I delivered wanted to go into the medical profession.

When older patients come in for gynecologic care, they usually have to wait for the obstetrical patients to be seen, and are, hopefully, patiently waiting in the reception area while their physician is delivering babies. Sometimes these women make a comment about waiting a long time, but usually they understand that the obstetrical patients come first. They remember that when they were pregnant, the doctor had to be readily available for deliveries and emergencies. Routine annual GYN examinations are usually a happy visit. The patient comes in to have an exam, get a Pap smear, schedule a mammogram, and discuss any concerns that have occurred over the last year. We update her medications, medical problems, and any surgery that may have taken place. About 75 percent of the time, I am that patient's only physician. In these cases, I refill any medication that she is taking on a regular basis and schedule any routine testing such as lab work, colonoscopies, cardiac evaluations, or immunizations. Gynecology patients tend to be older and the problems are different. Obstetrical patients worry all the time about eating the right things, avoiding foods and activities that may be harmful, worrying if there baby is moving enough, and if everything is going okay with the pregnancy. Gynecology patients (unless it is for an annual exam) are usually worried that they have an underlying problem (such as cancer), have a genital infection or pain, are depressed, have emotional problems, relationship problems, or have menopausal symptoms.

12
BUTTERFLIES

Many years ago I walked into a room and my high school physical education teacher was sitting in front of me. I loved her. She had the most precious, infectious laugh that I have ever heard in another human being. She was one of my favorite teachers in high school. It turned out that she was only about ten years older than I was. When you are in high school, the teachers always seem like they are so much older. In reality, many of them may be right out of college and in their student-teaching internships. It was early in my practice when she came to see me. I was about five years out of my residency, and obviously I did not have the self-confidence that I needed to take care of one of my former high school teachers. I know this, because it was another one of those times that I spoke without thinking.

I said, "I can't believe that you're going to let me take care of you." She looked at me with a very confused look on her face. She said, "Is there something I need to know about why you can't take care of me?" I said, "No, I just have never taken care of one of my teachers, and I was a little taken aback that one of my teachers would trust me to this degree." I learned a big lesson that day. No matter who is sitting in front of me, I must maintain my confidence in my abilities; it is important for the patient. When I teach medical students and residents, I always try to get this point across to them. At some point in their careers, they are going to take care of important people in the community, celebrities, former teachers, former professors, and others that you have looked up to your entire life. It is hard to get your hands around the fact that your roles have changed; someone who you looked up to your whole life now trusts you with theirs.

You must maintain your self-confidence. My physical education teacher whom I loved so much had breast cancer. It was a very early stage cancer. Although it was only stage 1, it was very aggressive. For some reason this early stage breast cancer kept recurring. She was going through chemotherapy for the third time when I first started taking care of her. I made it my mission in life to try to make her laugh. She obviously loved to laugh, but making her laugh was as much for me as it was for her. I took care of her for ten years before she died. I used to visit her in the hospital when she was getting chemotherapy. I was devastated when she died. Even worse, I missed the obituary in the paper and had not checked my e-mail for about a week because I was so busy. I completely missed the announcement of her death, and I missed her funeral. I can still hear her laugh in my head when I think about it.

About a year after her death, I found myself all alone on a beautiful Saturday afternoon. The children were at their grandparents' house, my husband was working at the hospital, and, mercifully, I was all alone at my own house. Women reading this will understand the beauty of being all alone in your own home with nobody needing you to take care of them. Those days are like gold and very rare. Normally I would have taken the opportunity to rush through the house like a mad woman cleaning, doing laundry, and tidying up. I decided that I was going to get a book, a novel, not a medical book or journal, and sit out by the pool. I was going to take a few hours for myself. The more I thought about it, the more excited I became. I was going to read a book next to the pool, all by myself, and not get disturbed, splashed, or asked to get up and make someone lunch. I even knew where I was going to put my chair. I am an avid gardener, and around my pool I had a raised planter full of zinnias. They were spectacular at this point of the year, and they were overflowing. I pushed a lounge chair up against the planter, which was about three feet high, put a towel down on the chair, and got a jug of ice-cold water and a glass beside me on the small table. The zinnias came down all around my head and surrounded me on both sides. I thanked God for my time alone, the beautiful day, and my flowers. I then promptly settled in my chair, picked up my romance novel, and started to read. Within thirty seconds a very large, beautiful orange butterfly settled on a flower right next to my face. It could not have been three inches from my eyes. Immediately upon looking at this butterfly, I knew that this butterfly represented my patient, my favorite teacher with the most wonderful laugh, telling me that she was okay, not hurting anymore, and was at peace. I was overwhelmed. It was the most peaceful feeling that I have ever encountered. I cried a little, both for my loss and for the honor of having this moment. I knew that Jesus was with me sitting on this lounge chair telling me that one of my favorite teachers, my patient, and my friend was okay.

I really thought that this moment was going to be short-lived. This butterfly, unbelievably, sat on this flower and never moved. After about thirty minutes of us looking at each other, I started to laugh a little bit. I could not believe that this overwhelming feeling of love and comfort was lasting this long. I wanted to get a picture of this butterfly so that I could always remember this moment, but I really thought that as soon as I got up, the butterfly would leave. Eventually I did get up, went into the house, and got a camera. When I came out, the butterfly was still sitting on the same flower. I took some pictures from several angles and then slowly sat back down in my lounge chair. I took more pictures sitting in the chair within inches of the butterfly. When I was finished taking pictures, I put down the camera, looked back at the butterfly and said, "Thank you for this moment." With that, the butterfly flew away. Several months later I took several rolls of film in to the store to be developed.

When I picked up the film, I sat in my car to look at the pictures that I thought were only of my children. I was surprised to open up one of the packages and find my butterfly pictures. They were beautiful; they were peaceful. I went back into the photo store and got one more set of the butterfly pictures. I then went to Walmart and picked up two frames. That night I made two collages of the butterfly pictures. I hung one up in my office and saved the other one for my patient's family. My dilemma, now, was how I was going to explain my collage to this family that I had never met without them thinking that I was a complete nut ball. Embarrassingly, I held onto that picture and never contacted the family. I was just too uncomfortable.

About two years later I walked into an examination room to see a new patient. After I introduced myself, reviewed her chart, and examined her, I asked her if there was anything else that she would like to discuss. She said, "No, but I would like you to know that my sister-in-law was your patient and she talked about how much she loved having you as her doctor. When I needed a new gynecologist, I knew that I would come to you." I asked her the name of her sister-in-law. Shocked and stunned to find out that it was my patient and former teacher, I sat down and became tearful.

My patient was now comforting me. I told her that I loved her sister-in-law very much and that over the years we had become friends. I looked at her and said, "I need to tell you a story." I proceeded to tell her the story of my wonderful afternoon alone by the pool. I told her that I was a little embarrassed to tell her about how strongly I felt that her sister-in-law personified this butterfly. I do not believe in reincarnation at all, and I do not believe that her family member "came back" as a butterfly. I told her that I did believe that Jesus made me think of her as that beautiful butterfly. I told her that I would like to give her the collage that I made. She said, "That is so appropriate because of the butterflies." I looked at her and said, "What do you mean?" She said, "Weren't you at the funeral?" I told her how upset I had been when I found out about her death after her funeral. She looked at me in shock and said, "You mean, you don't know about the butterflies?" I looked at her in bewilderment. She started to cry a little too. She said that she loved butterflies more than anything in the world and that her students all knew how much she loved them. She taught school up until her death. At her funeral all the students from Savannah Christian Preparatory School made cards in the shape of butterflies. There were hundreds of butterflies all over the pews of the church and all over her casket.

Godwink.

Her family now has the collage that I made.

13
A Genital Handywoman

As with any surgical specialty, you get more comfortable as you do more and more surgeries. When you first get out of your residency, an OB/GYN's primary surgical procedure is a cesarean section. Because obstetrics is your primary focus as a young OB/GYN, you are going to encounter more patients needing a cesarean section than a hysterectomy. Gynecology is a fix-it specialty; we are always fixing something that is not working correctly or removing something that is not supposed to be there. For instance, if your uterus is bleeding too much (or causing you pain), we take it out. If you have abnormal cells on your vulva, vagina, or cervix, we cut them out. If your bladder, rectum, or uterus is falling out, we tack it up. If you have a mass on your uterus, fallopian tubes, or on your ovaries, we remove them. If you cannot get pregnant, we look in your pelvis to see what is wrong.

Most of our surgery is "quality-of-life" surgery; it is performed to improve your quality of life. Quality-of-life surgery is different from elective surgery. You cannot just have a GYN surgery because you want one. You have to have a good indication to have the surgery and have to have tried some conservative methods to fix your problem. On the other hand, except for taking out an abnormal ovary or a suspicion of cancer, if you are not medically able to withstand the surgery, you are probably not going to have it. For example, if you are eighty years old, and you have severe coronary heart disease and go to your OB/GYN with your bladder falling out, you are probably going to die with your bladder falling out. It is just not a surgical emergency. I agree that it is profoundly annoying. It is annoying for you and for your caretaker, but under most circumstances, it is not going to hurt you. This statement is in no way meant to be mean or cruel.

Remember how I explained the "second victim" in the practice of obstetrics? This also applies to gynecology. Sometimes an OB/GYN encounters a patient who comes in with their family and begs for her bladder to be "tacked up" in her vagina. They tell you that they will sign a waiver that they will not hold you accountable for her death or blame you for her death if something were to happen during the surgery. There is no doubt that the patient does not want to live anymore with her problem; however, the family and the patient fail to realize that the physician is also a participant in the decision. The physician will be devastated if their patient dies from a surgery that was not indicated to save their patient's life.

There are two people in the "doctor-patient" relationship. How would you feel if you did something to someone and knew that there was a chance that the person would die if you did it (even though it was to help them), and then they died? This situation was presented to me recently when my husband and I went out to dinner with another couple. The husband of the other couple told me that his ninety-eight-year-old aunt was in the ICU after a severe heart attack. One of the doctors taking care of her mentioned that if she were younger, she could have benefited from bypass surgery. He asked the doctor why she could not have it at her age. The doctor said that there was a very high chance that she would not make it through the surgery. The man went on and on complaining to me that it does not matter what age someone was, the surgeon should try the surgery to see if it worked. I said, "And what if you were the doctor? How would you feel if you operated on someone knowing that they had a 98 percent chance of dying from the surgery, and the person died? If she did not have the surgery, there was still a good chance that she could be managed with medication. Medical management of the situation is the best option." He looked at me and said, "I never thought about what the doctor felt." I know.

14
FRIENDSHIP

I moved into my house on Whitemarsh Island in October 2003. It was a great house on a cul-de-sac. The children were five years old, and while I was unpacking, a great friend of mine walked in the door with a plate of brownies. She said, "I live two houses down, and we are so glad that you are here." She and I were pregnant together and had known each other since 1992, when I had interviewed for a residency in Savannah. She was a Labor and Delivery nurse, and I loved her. We had both had been previously married, and we both married older men who had had a previous family. We both were stepmothers to two older children, and we both had five step-grandchildren. Everything was perfect. Our husbands became good friends; our children became "best" friends.

About two and a half years later, our families were staying at a beach house at Tybee Island. The children were downstairs playing, and we were upstairs having some adult beverages and telling stories. We started talking about our friendship and that it meant so much to us all. It was a very emotional conversation. It was a conversation that, at the time, I knew was going be one of those important memories. Unexpectedly my friend's husband said, "This friendship is more important than you remember."

He then got up and sat on the ottoman in front of my husband. He grabbed his hands, brought them together with his, and held them. He said, "You don't remember me, but I remember you. As you know, I had another life before this marriage. You do not remember my first wife. I am older now, gray-haired, wear glasses, and have put on some weight so there is no reason for you to remember me. My wife and I lived in South Georgia, and we traveled up to Augusta to the Medical College of Georgia to see you. She had ovarian cancer, and you took care of her." My husband had this look of embarrassment and concern, and I knew that he felt bad that he did not remember them. As he started to apologize, my friend's husband quieted him and said, "You took care of my wife and me as if we were your only patients in the world. You treated us as if we had all the money in the world. I will never forget or be able to repay your kindness. I just want you to know that I am honored to be your friend. It is one of the most meaningful friendships of my life." Well, you could have seen four people crying and holding each other.

Godwink.

It was one of those moments.

15
CANCER, GODWINKS, FRIENDS, AND FAMILY

I stopped delivering babies "officially" on December 31, 2006. In 2005 my husband developed a rare cancer of the minor salivary glands under his jawbone. It was a terrible two years trying to take night call, see patients in the office, operate, and take care of my family. My twins were eight years old. They were participating in many sports and school events. I had a nanny, but it was difficult to manage it all. I look back now and realize that I should have quit obstetrics earlier, but I kept thinking that it was all going to get better. I thought that my life would go back to the way it used to be. It didn't.

My husband had ten surgeries from 2005 through 2006. He was scheduled for another. It just was not getting any better; in fact, I thought that it was getting worse. I really wanted to get a second opinion; however, that is very difficult when both the patient and the spouse are physicians. We did not want to offend his doctors. They loved and cared for both of us. I really think that I was as close to what was a nervous breakdown as I could get. I was so tired, worried, scared, and overwhelmed. On one particular evening, I got home late and drove down my street. My husband was in pain, and he had called me wondering where I was and when I was coming home. I ran into the house. He was yelling for pain medication, the children were hungry and crying, the nanny was saying goodbye, and the phone was ringing. I answered the phone; it was my friend two doors down. She told me that she really needed me at her house for a minute. She asked if I could come right over. I quickly ran down the street and she met me at the front door. She grabbed my hand and pulled me into her kitchen. There was a steak and baked potato with a large glass of milk in front of me. She told me that I was too thin and that I was not eating. She told me to finish eating, and then I could go right home. I resigned myself to try to calmly eat and not think about the disaster that I had left at the house. She got up, and her husband sat down. He said, "Your husband helped my family get through the death of my wife, and I will never forget that as long as I live. I have a private plane, and I just want you to know that if you need to go to any other medical center in the world, I will take you all there." I thanked him and told him that I did not think that we were going anywhere, but I would keep it in mind. I ran back home and took care of my family. The next day, I ran into my husband's doctor in the hallway. He came right up to me, grabbed my hands, and said, "I know that we have surgery scheduled for two days from now, but I think it is time to get out of Savannah. We cannot really handle his case here anymore, and I do not think that anyone here wants to admit it." It's hard to take care of another doctor.

Godwink.

I respected his honesty more than he would ever know. I told him that. He asked me if I knew anyone in Houston because MD Anderson Cancer Center in Houston, Texas, was where we should go. My husband's colleague and closest friend lived in Houston. He was a doctor. I called him and asked him if he could pull some strings and get my dying husband into see someone in the Ear, Nose, and Throat (ENT) department as soon as possible. He called me back an hour later and said that the chairman of ENT could see him at 10:30 the next morning. He said, "I know it seems impossible, but can you get here?"

Godwink.

I think that I can.

I cancelled all of my patients for the week and drove home. I got out of the car and for the second time in two days ran down the street to my friend's house. I rang the doorbell, and almost immediately her husband opened the door. Through a flood of tears, I said, "I think I need your plane." He took the information from me and told me to go home and start packing. He would call me back in fifteen minutes. Exactly fifteen minutes later, the phone rang with instructions for the next morning. At 5:30 the next morning, we were at a private airport with clothes for all four of us for two weeks. We had all of the medical equipment, intravenous fluids, and food for tube feeding. The pilot and I packed the plane, and we took off. I prayed the whole way to Houston that my husband would not die in front of the children on the plane. We landed in Houston at 9 A.M. A car drove out to the plane when it stopped, and four men got out and helped us all into the car. I later found out that none of them worked there; they were just pilots that were sitting in the airport waiting to leave and heard on the radio that we would need help. They rode out to the plane in the rented car with the person from the rental car place so that my husband would not have to walk. The pilot came over to my window and handed me his card. He said, "Go to your appointment. I will be here waiting for you. If they cannot help him, I will be here to take you home. If they can help him and you can stay, then I will come back with the plane to get you. You have many people praying for you." I drove to the appointment. At 4:30 P.M., after CT scans and testing, the chair of the ENT department said that he wanted to try to operate. He scheduled surgery for the next day. I called the pilot back. He said, "Just call me, and I will come back to pick you up. We will all be here when you need us."

We stayed in Houston, Texas, at the house of my husband's friend for a month. They helped us so much with the children. However, I could not wait to go home. When I got home, I found that my friend had cleaned my whole house, cleaned out the fridge, and made us dinner. I cannot describe what an act of kindness that was. My husband lived another five years. He would not have made it if we had not gone to that medical center. Many people helped to save his life, and I will be forever grateful. We were working on our Christmas cards the night before he died. As usual, we were late getting them out. He had had another recurrence of his cancer a few months earlier, and like the last recurrence, they gave him some more radiation to "try to control it." It worked for a little while. The worst thing for my husband was admitting that he was sick. His only goal was to work and let the kids have as normal a life as possible. He did both. He worked up until the week before he died. The last thing that he did was operate with his OB/GYN residents. He then saw a couple of patients who were in his office. He had been coughing terribly for months; however, the last two weeks were just awful. I do not think that he ever really slept. He would only take short naps before the coughing would come back. The doctors decided to try some chemotherapy, and he got his first infusion on January 7, 2011. I went and sat with him while he got the chemotherapy, and he was in a good mood. We left, picked up my daughter from basketball practice, and went home. We worked on our Christmas cards. My son had left school at noon that day with his wrestling coach to go to a multi-school wrestling tournament in Dublin, Georgia. The other parents on the team kept texting us with his wins and updates on the tournament. We were cheering in the living room because he was winning every match. My husband was so proud of him. We wished that we could have been there to watch him. We were waiting up for the coach to call us when they got back into Savannah, and I was going to go pick him up at their house. To our surprise, the coach pulled into our driveway at midnight with my son grinning from ear-to-ear. The coach wanted to be with our son and see our faces when he told us that he was voted "Most Outstanding Wrestler" of the whole tournament. He had a large wall plaque that we could put a picture in and hang on the wall. My husband was overwhelmed with pride. My children went to bed that night hearing their father saying repeatedly how much he loved them. He told them that he was proud of both of them. He told my son that there was never a day in his life that he had ever been more proud of him. We had a big family kiss and hug, and then the kids went to bed laughing and happy. When he finally stopped coughing about 3 A.M., he got into bed and said, "Promise me that you love me." I said, "I promise you that I love you." He said, "That is all I need to know."

He was gone when I woke up. He did not want to stop working, and he did not. He did not want to lose his hair because the kids might be scared, and he did not. He did not want people to know how sick he was, and for the most part, they did not. If you were a colleague, the feelings and admiration that you had for him were mutual. If you were a patient, he loved and cared for you as much as you loved and cared for him. For his friends, and especially his family, there were no words to describe how he felt about you. You were loved more than anything in the world. If you were his resident, he loved you as much as you loved him, and he loved teaching you more than you loved him to teach you. He was a great physician and father. He loved Miller Lite more than I love Budweiser. When it rains I visualize him popping a beer with Jesus, and the rain is just the foam falling over their beer glasses.

16
GYNECHIATRY

In January 2007 I found myself with no obstetrical patients and not having to run to Labor and Delivery anymore. All of a sudden I was in the office all the time and had more time to spend with each patient. When I had a large obstetrical load, the practice of gynecology was seeing patients with problems and subsequently operating on them to fix those problems. It is so much more. When I was doing obstetrics, I never had time to put my whole heart and soul into gynecology. I really had to learn many new things. I had to learn a completely new way of practicing medicine. Obstetrics visits are quick, fun, and to the point; gynecology visits are long, sometimes sad, and never to the point. It takes quite a long time for patients to get to the comfort level during the visit to tell you what they really want to tell you. What is an OB/GYN called that does not practice obstetrics anymore? A "gynechiatrist."

Sometimes I think that one of the most important aspects of the gynecologic visit is listening. I never realized how difficult it is to learn to listen. I can remember the first day of medical school and the professor saying to us that on average a physician interrupts their patient within twelve seconds of walking into the room. He said that if we would listen (and not talk) for two minutes, the patient would tell you what is wrong with them. The patient would be most happy because you took the time to listen. Sometimes it is extremely hard to sit and listen for two minutes.

The psychiatry part of gynecology works both ways. Sometimes the patient helps me get through things as much as I help them. Listening to stories from my patients about what is happening to them in their lives gives me time to think about what is happening in my life. For instance, if someone is going through a horrible time with her husband or children, not only am I in awe that she is handling problems with courage and finesse, but I also see that my life is not as difficult as I thought. I think that this happens to everyone. If you take the time to sit down and talk with someone (even someone you know very well), you will learn that they have trials and tribulations in their lives that are significant as well. We all have significant challenges, disappointments, and trials. Most of the time we are so self-absorbed in our own problems that we do not look around and see that it may not be as bad as we think.

I can think of one patient in particular. She is in her mid-fifties and has had more challenges in her life than most of us will ever encounter. She had been diagnosed with stage III ovarian cancer fifteen years ago. She is one of the few patients that I know who has lived this long after this diagnosis. Bizarrely, several years later, she was in the wrong place at the wrong time and sustained a gunshot wound to her head resulting in the loss of vision in one eye. She has frequently pondered her life and luck while we were talking during her annual examinations. She frequently would end the conversation with the words, "God has a purpose for my life. He must, because there is no reason for me to be here." This year our conversation changed. I walked into the examination room to perform her annual exam, and this elegant, highly educated, and, what would seem like, very unlucky woman started the conversation by telling me that Jesus had finally revealed the reason why she survived all of her trials. During the prior few years, her son had been living with a woman who had a baby from a previous relationship. Her son had been with this woman since her baby was one month old. Two years later they had their own child, and my patient was the loving grandmother to these two beautiful girls. Unfortunately, her son and the girl's mother ended up with a significant drug habit. She and her husband were given custody of the girls. My patient told me this story through tears of joy, wonderment, and peace. She said, "Jesus let me live so that I could take care of these two girls and bring them up in a loving, stable home. I hope that my husband and I live long enough to see them through until they are old enough to take care of themselves." I have a feeling that they will.

There are many funny things that happen in gynecology; most of the time, it is not funny when it is happening, but when you look back, it is hysterical. I remember one woman in particular who had bad back pain. She had been to multiple physicians and found that the narcotic Percocet really helped her back pain. I am sure it was good for her back pain, but it is unethical to keep prescribing that strong of a narcotic on a regular basis. Percocet is a highly addictive drug and you have to be careful about how much you prescribe. The physicians in my practice have an office policy that we only give narcotics for postoperative pain. We do not give narcotics for chronic pain of any type. For this type of chronic pain, a patient should really see a pain specialist and sign a contract with that physician to limit their use of narcotics. However, it is hard to look at someone in front of you who is obviously in pain and not give them something to help them. After the first time she saw me, I did give her some Percocet until she could get in to see a pain specialist. I did make sure that she had the appointment and that the girls at the front desk reminded her of the time and date.

I was surprised when she came back to see me two weeks later with a giant bag of Vidalia onions. She handed me the bag and promptly asked for a refill of Percocet until the visit with the pain specialist. I explained the office policy about narcotics to my patient and told her that the first prescription was supposed to last her until she met with the specialist. She said, "But I brought you a bag of onions!" I said, "I appreciate it, but you cannot give me onions for a Percocet prescription. Besides, what am I going to do with that many onions?" Seeing a possibility that I might change my mind, she quickly said, "I'll bring you back some recipes." Sorry.

I walked into one room and my patient was looking very angry. She had her lips pursed, her legs crossed, and she was swinging her leg up and down quickly. I looked at her and immediately thought that I must be really far behind in my schedule, because she was angry. I looked at the clock and saw that it was not too bad, and I asked her if she was angry with me. I was thinking that perhaps one of the girls in the office had been rude to her, or perhaps we had gotten her bill incorrect, or that she wanted to talk about it. Before I could verbalize any of this, she looked at me and said, "I have a small home office. It is really just a large closet; the office has a desk, file cabinet, trashcan, computer, and printer. When it is cold outside, I am usually in there with the door shut and my dog at my feet. My husband came home today and opened the door to my office. He was talking to me, but as he was talking, he was looking around this small room and even looked in my trashcan and opened the file cabinets. He looked at me, sniffed, and asked me where the fish was in the room. She said, "Doctor, I need you to find the fish and get rid of it." Don't worry, I got this.

17
CHEATING AND STRAYING

Many times in the office women come in to talk because they are going through a divorce. I am a very safe person to talk to about this issue. Everything is completely confidential, I can give advice, and they do not have to worry that what they are going to tell me will ever come back and haunt them. If you tell your best friend something terrible (such as, your husband is beating you), and you decide to stay with him, she will always know that you put up with that. You will always wonder what she really thinks of you. With me, there is a small chance that she has to worry about me thinking badly of her. Most of the time I am out of sight and out of mind until her next visit. When a husband is cheating, I know immediately because my patient starts crying very hard when I open the door. She is angry about the affair and scared that she may have contracted something. Sometimes the woman is cheating, actually "straying." I have learned through the years that men "cheat" and women "stray." Even when they are the ones that go outside the marriage, they are still worried that they have contracted a sexually transmitted disease. One patient said it particularly well: "I took a bite of the outside cheese, and it was moldy."

18
NAMES

There are times when, as a surgeon, you realize that people do not really know their anatomy. Even when you think you are using terms that are not "medical," some of my patients still do not exactly know what I really am going to do to them in surgery. It is very important to make sure that the patient understands exactly what is going to be removed or repaired. One day I realized that my patient had heard the word hysterectomy, but was not exactly sure what was going to be taken out of her. I finally realized that she understood when she said, "I get it! You are going to take the gift and leave the box."

I am not sure if people in other parts of the country refer to their genitals with special words, but in the South we have some special names. For example, the area between the vaginal opening and the anus (the perineum) is called "the taint." T'aint your vagina and t'aint your ass. It is "the taint." Women come in all the time with "itching on my taint." The labia majora, or the larger, outer lips, are frequently referred to as "mud-flaps." For example, "Doctor, my mud-flaps are itching again," or "I looked with a mirror and one of my mud-flaps is larger than the other. Is that normal?" If you live in the South and have ever gone mud-boggin, you know the importance of mud-flaps. Men may call a vagina a "pussy," but you know that a Southern woman would *never* say that word. Now, we might just refer to that special area as "the cat." For example, "Honey, I am going to take the cat to the vet. I'll be back in a few hours." Alternatively, you might hear, "I'm going to put the cat in the shower so that she'll be nice and fresh for the vet." If we are talking about something sexual, we might refer to that special place as "the kitty." For example, "Doctor, my kitty doesn't feel good because she has had a fever lately." Translation: My vagina has been getting a lot of action lately, and I think that I may have caught something. Sometimes a woman comes in and says, "I'm having 'Hello Kitty' problems." Another very funny line that a woman used was, "Doctor, I used to have the cleanest kitty in Liberty County, but some alcohol was added and bad decisions were made. I need to get her clean again." Don't worry, I got this. Women also have names for their period. It is just as likely for a woman to tell me that she had to cancel her last two appointments because it was her "lady time," as it is to hear, "I came in because 'Demonica' is here again this month, and she is hurting me badly." If there are any men out there who are shaking their heads and laughing after reading this last paragraph, please give us a break. There is not a woman in the world who has not heard their partner's special name for their penis.

19
THE SPECULUM

Over the years many women have asked me about the "speculum," which is the metal or plastic device that is inserted inside the vagina in order to see the cervix or do a pap smear. Most of them make a comment that a man must have invented it because they do not like having it put inside them. Actually this clever little device has been perfected over the years. The earliest recorded evidence of the speculum is in the Talmud about 1300 B.C. (800 years before Hippocrates). This was a cylinder made from bamboo or from the stem of a gourd. Clever.

There is controversy over whether Hippocrates used a speculum or a "mitroscope," which was similar to the duckbilled speculum of the nineteenth century. The first record of a speculum was by Galen (A.D. 130–200). In 1818 two specula were found in the excavations of Pompeii that had to have been buried since A.D. 79. Soranus (A.D. 98–177) wrote an entire chapter on the speculum in his book of gynecology. Aetius in the sixth century and Aegina (sounds like vagina?) in the seventh century used a cylindrical type of speculum. Aluscasis in 1085 described specula of ebony and boxwood. Paré (1510–1590) talked of the speculum when he discussed visualizing cervical cancer. Marie Anne Victoire Bolvin (1773–1841) was a very famous and well-educated midwife in Paris. She came up with the idea for the bivalve vaginal speculum in 1825. James Marion Sims (1813–1883) founded the first American hospital devoted to gynecology in 1855. He developed a speculum that we still use today: the Sims Speculum. There is a bronze statue of Dr. Sims in Central Park, New York. Sir William Fergusson of London used a tubular speculum in 1870. This speculum consisted of a cylindrical tube of glass coated with mercury, covered with India rubber, and thoroughly varnished throughout. It was considered the best, the most useful and cleanest speculum in its day.

A man named Martin invented a bath speculum in the latter part of the nineteenth century that was a vaginal dilator introduced during a bath to allow inward bathing of the vagina. Why did a man develop a speculum to be used in a bathtub? See, people were kinky back then, too.

In addition, why was this so important to him? I would have hated to have been his wife, because, it could be assumed that he made it because her vagina smelled badly. I would have killed him. It is reported that this speculum never became popular. I cannot imagine why not.

Just so that I do not offend those gynecologists of old, the others that modified or tried to perfect the speculum were Reuff, Astruc, Recamier, Dupuytren, Osiander, Ricord, Eegales, Charriere, Cusco, Brewer, Bozeman, Collins, Goodell, Hirst, Erskine, Graves, Stallworthy, and Ashurst. Women should give extra "kudos" to Ashurst, who in his book, in 1889, described the use of the speculum in the following manner: "The speculum should always be introduced well-warmed and oiled, under cover of the patient's garments of bed clothes, without any exposure of the person." How nice!

He must have been a very gentle and compassionate man. I probably would have gone to him. If you ever got to look at pictures of the specula of old, you would be thankful for the ones that we have now.

Therefore, I have answered my patient's questions. I report to you that there were many men who invented the speculum, and one brilliant woman who was a midwife from Paris, France. One woman was involved. There ya go.

20
HOLES AND HAIR

As I indicated earlier, people ask me all the time how I chose gynecology. I tell them how I fell in love with the babies and the gynecology fell in behind. However, people ask all kinds of questions about my day. They are not being rude, and I never take it as a rude question; I believe they are genuinely interested and curious about what it is I do. One of my favorite questions is, "Do you ever look at your schedule in the morning, and say, 'God, I can't stand one more vagina in my office this week'?" No, I really don't.

There are also questions such as, "How could you spend your whole day looking at other women's vaginas? I don't even like to look at my pubic hair!" It is different when you are helping someone feel better. To me, it is just like looking at your arm all day. The comment about the pubic hair reminds me of a patient that I had who was in graduate school at the Savannah College of Art and Design (SCAD). She was a graduate student in film and asked if she could come to the office with some of her classmates and interview me on a topic while filming me. I told her that would be okay and that she should schedule it with the receptionist. Really, I forgot about it. One day, however, I had finished early and was thinking that several people must have canceled. I started to walk up to the front desk to see if I was finished for the day when the receptionist turned around, looked at me, and said, "You are not going to believe this." I looked out into the waiting room and saw four large television cameras and my patient with a microphone. I thought this might be fun, it was a break from the monotony of the week, and I really would be helping my patient with her project. I walked out into the waiting room. The students thanked me for participating with their project. I told them that I was happy to do so and asked how we should start. My patient told me that she was just going to start asking me questions, and I was to try to act as if the cameras were not in the room. She proceeded to interview me at length about pubic hair. I was shocked out of my mind, but I did not want them to think that this was bothering me. Therefore, I gave them all the answers that they requested and talked more about pubic hair in that hour than I ever have in my life. I was asked about the percentage of women who shaved their pubic hair, the designs that I have seen, the designs that I liked, and the designs that were surprising. I told them that the most surprising design was of a target: like a bull's-eye. I was surprised because I had never seen anything like that, and I thought that it must take an incredible amount of time to maintain. I would never have that much time to devote to maintaining something like that.

After they were finished, they asked if I had any questions for them. My first question was about what they were going to do with the film. I calmed down a little when they promised me that it would go no further than their class. I told them that if I ever ran for president of the United States, I had better not see that film. They promised. I am not sure when it became common practice for women to shave their pubic hair. I can remember seeing this for the first time as an OB/GYN resident in 1990. A girl came into Labor and Delivery completely shaved. The nurse gasped and said, "Honey, you really don't have to shave your hair to have a baby anymore." She looked at her boyfriend and smiled a very mischievous smile. She said, "He likes it when I shave it bald." He nodded and said, "I like the feel of it with no hair on it." The nurse walked out of the room and, as she passed us, she whispered that he was probably a pedophile. After that, it became more and more common; and at some point, it seemed like everybody was shaving. Now my patients come in and are embarrassed if they have not shaved. They apologize because they are not "appropriately groomed" for the visit. Don't worry, I didn't shave for you either.

One of my patients was getting her exam and, as instructed, came down to the bottom of the table and put her feet up into stirrups. When I pulled the sheet back, she had a Post-it note stuck to her pubic hair that said, "Sorry, the landscaper is gone for the winter." Very cute. No problem.

The question of pubic-hair shaving comes up a lot in the office. Women would like to know what other women are doing. I would guess that about 65 percent of women shave some or all of their pubic hair. The external genitalia have very sensitive tissues. I always tell young girls to pick one brand of soap and stay with it for your entire life. When I talk to young pre-pubertal girls about puberty, I tell them to Dove their dove. Have your mom get Dove Sensitive Skin soap and only buy that brand for washing your private parts. I do not care what fancy, wonderful smelling bath soaps and gels that you get for the rest of your body, always stick to one brand for the dove. Most women are acutely aware of this as we have all received bath gels at Christmas or for birthday gifts and promptly got a rash and itching. It is important not to switch laundry detergents also. The changing of chemicals and scents that touch the genitalia can cause a significant irritation. I was told in medical school that the pubic hair protects the opening of the vagina from infections. That does not seem to have been true because the majority of women seem to shave and there really is not an increase in infections (from my point of view, anyway). Does shaving cause any problems? Some women get "shave bumps" and ingrown hairs from shaving the labia. Besides being a little annoying, it does not appear to hurt anything. There are several ways to remove the hair from the labia. The most popular method is shaving with a razor. Many women get the hair pulled out with hot wax. It evidently hurts terribly, but the hair stays gone for a longer period. Laser hair removal is becoming more and more popular. The initial investment is large, but you may never have to shave again. There are various depilatory creams and lotions. These are not as popular, and many women come in with significant reactions to the chemicals.

I do have a story about waxing that may make you stop waxing. I had a patient that was at her salon getting a wax. She had never done it before, so as you can imagine, she was extremely nervous. The employees at the salon were extremely nice to her, comforted her, and were there to hold her hand throughout the entire procedure. She relaxed and calmed down. The young woman pulled off the linen that covered the hot wax, and her entire labia majora ripped open. I was not there, but evidently it looked like someone was killed. They had never seen so much blood at one time. She came by ambulance to the hospital, got two units of blood, and we sutured it closed in the operating room. I do not think that she is going to do it again.

As you get older, pubic hair turns gray after menopause and falls out. This is something that people ask me about all the time. They are worried that they are not normal. They are normal.

21
Tattoos and Tales From the Table

Talking about pubic hair makes me think of other things that people do to their genital region. Piercings are very common in this area of the body, and I am actually shocked that people do not ask their gynecologist to put these piercings into their labia and clitoris with some local anesthesia. I would ask my gynecologist to do this before I ever let a man in a tattoo parlor put one in my labia or clitoris. I would probably do it for them just so they would not do it in a tattoo parlor. However, I have never been asked to do this. I walked into another exam room and the patient yelled, "Hey doc! I have three new friends!" I looked at her, and she was naked. She was spread eagle on the table, and had three new vulvar piercings. She had one in her clitoral hood and one in each of her labia. She said, "Trust me. If you get your clitoris pierced you will get a motorcycle. I bought a motorcycle and I ride around town happy and screaming with delight!" Another girl, very seriously, wanted me to know that she put her Harley Davidson clitoral ring on just for me. It was a special occasion. It was a great compliment to me, because it meant a lot to her. I was a "Harley worthy" doctor. Breast barbells are another piercing that I see often. With the number of nerve endings in the nipple, I do not understand how it is not terribly painful. I asked one woman specifically about them. She said, "I like them, but it is so expensive." I thought that maybe it was expensive initially to put them in, but, after it is done, there should be no expense. She said, "That's how it should be, but my husband keeps swallowing them, and I have to keep buying new ones." Hickeys are another thing that I find on the breasts regularly. One woman said it best when she saw me looking at about twenty of them. She said, "He was a bad boy and I had a good time!"

As you can imagine, alcohol plays a significant role in people making bad decisions and needing my services. For example, "Doctor, I had stupid tequila sex. Can you make sure that I am okay?" Another example was actually scary for the whole office. The receptionist transferred a phone call to me, and my patient said, "Doctor, I have been drinking. I cannot find my husband's head. I am calling the police. I thought that you should know." Click (phone went dead). That was a bad call. Yes, we did keep trying to call her; and no, she never picked the phone back up that day. Her husband came by the next day and told us that he was sorry about the phone call. He explained that they had had a fight. Ya think?

One younger patient came in and asked me about the condoms that she bought. She was under age (for drinking alcohol), and she handed me the condom pack to inspect. There was a warning on this "whiskey-flavored" condom: "Do not use while driving." She wanted to know if it was legal for her to have bought them. I wanted to know why the authorities are so worried about people talking on their phones while driving. I said, "Where do you buy these?" www.heritageof-scotland.com.

There is a new flavor of condoms in town. Whiskey-flavored. Ideal for that special woman or man in your life who likes more than their liquor hard. Also perfect for when you need to stop that more casual someone, from sobering up. I can't make this stuff up.

I took care of one patient who needed a hysterectomy. She was in a hot and heavy new romance. Both of them had been divorced for many years and really thought that they would always be alone. Their story was so wonderful. He came to all of her preoperative appointments with her and asked very appropriate questions. The problem was that even in the office they could not keep their hands off each other. I gave them the postoperative instructions and looked both of them in the eyes. I said, "You cannot have intercourse until the four-week postoperative checkup. I want to see the top of the vagina and make sure that it is healed." They laughed and assured me that they had already discussed it, and they planned to do "other things." Perfect. Two days later I was urgently called to the emergency room and was very upset to see her in a bed. She and her partner were holding hands and crying. He was crying particularly hard. Neither one of them would look at me. Once I had closed the door, and still without looking at me, she lifted the sheet up. There, between the sheets, were some of her intestines. They had covered them up to her vagina in a Ziploc bag. We went back to the operating room immediately. She did fine. It is funny now.

22
LAUGHTER, LOVE, AND DIVINE INTERVENTION

After my husband died on January 8, 2011, I had to sell my house. My husband made a lot more money than I did, and we had a large house on Whitemarsh Island and a beach house at Tybee. I could not afford to keep all of this property, so I decided to put it all on the market. We would live in whichever house did not sell. The house on Whitemarsh Island sold first, which was only 3.6 miles from my office (talk about convenience). However, our church was at Tybee, and we had wonderful memories of our family at the beach. Before we moved I sat my children down and told them that we were not going to make any big decisions. I was going to concentrate on three things: going to church, getting them through high school and into college (they were in the eighth grade), and work. I had put the life insurance money in an account for their college. I was hoping not to touch it; I wanted to live on my salary alone. Therefore, we started moving to Tybee Island. My children were furious with me. They wanted to stay, and I understood their emotions completely. I tried to explain that they would be teenagers living at the beach. They did not want to leave their friends; I tried to explain that their friends would come to them. I was informed by my children that I did not understand their generation.

One Sunday morning when we were leaving church, my daughter got into my truck and slammed the door. A disgusted statement directed towards me accompanied this. In that thirteen-year-old girl voice, she said, "You are humiliating." What? Oh No! I was having such a nice morning! It was a beautiful summer day, and I had just been admiring the flowers around the church. I looked at her and said, "What now?" She said, "You are humiliating. You and the man in front of you talk the whole service, and everybody notices, even the priest." Well, you have to understand our little church. There are only about ten pews on each side of the aisle. Because my children were serving at the altar with the priest during the service, my late husband and I sat on the second pew. They were very young when they started participating in the service; they were acolytes. They carried the candles or the cross to the front of the church and helped with communion. They started doing this when they were about six years old. I was a little nervous about it at first, but they were the only age-appropriate children in the congregation at the time. Therefore, we sat up front to keep our eyes on them. Sometimes they would start fighting up on the altar or begin laughing at each other. Sometimes my son would start twirling the cross or they would blow out the candles, then look at us, and mouth the words, "I didn't mean to do it." After my husband died, I just kept my seat on the second pew. They really did not need supervision anymore, but it was my usual seat. No one ever sat with me because they all had their own pew to sit on. This probably happens in other churches too, but in our Episcopal Church everyone stays on their own pew. This man would come in and sit on the front pew by himself, and I was on the second pew by myself. It was funny that no one ever sat next to me. We started talking to each other. When my daughter told me that everyone in the church was looking at me, I realized that this could be true. Everyone was sitting behind me, and my children were on the altar looking out at the congregation. I got this very horrified look on my face and said, "Really?" She said, "Yes, it is humiliating." Just when I started to rationalize this away by realizing that a thirteen-year-old girl was saying this, my son said, "It is humiliating Mom; don't you notice the priest looking at you two when you are talking?" I did not know how to respond. I could feel my face turning red and hot. The next week in church, I told this man about the conversation with my children. He said, "I'll move back to the second pew."

We got married a year later. We invited a few close friends to the wedding in addition to our immediate families. We also invited our church family. The priest gave a beautiful sermon about how everyone in the church knew that our finding each other had to be divine intervention. Someone in the back yelled, "We knew it was over when he moved to the second pew." Everyone laughed. My best friend and her family came to my wedding; she gave me a giant salt block as a wedding present. You can use it as a cutting board for cooking, and you can put it on the grill and cook your steak right on the salt block. The salt flavor infuses into everything that you cook on the block. You have to understand that salt is my favorite food. My second favorite food is cheese grits. I think that the only reason that I love cheese grits is so that I can put salt on them. The salt block was a perfect gift. It was from a friend who knows everything about me. I love her.

23
Faith and Fun

I talk a lot about my faith in the office, so my patients know that I am a Christian. I pray with people all the time about their situations and challenges. It is common for a patient to tell me about her spiritual experiences. One woman jumped off the table when I walked into the room and shouted, "I have proof that there is a God. My husband was getting a vasectomy, and, after he was undressed and draped on the procedure table, they brought me in to hold his hand. They put his feet up in stirrups. He looked at me and whispered, 'They are under the drape working. I can't see what they are doing! Can you believe this'?" She's right. She has proof. Men sometimes come into the office with their wives or girlfriends. They are usually very uncomfortable. It does not help that I have signs all over the walls about how God made the rough draft (men) before he made the masterpiece (women). There is a paperback in each room with the title "The World's Stupidest Men." This book has a bunch of short stories about stupid things that men do. My patients are always asking me if they can get a copy of a page or two before they leave, because the stories are so funny. When a man comes into the exam room, I usually make a comment that they are in a place of honor in the "inner sanctum" of the office (the examination room) and that sometimes men were never seen or heard from again. I remember one man who was completely comfortable. I had recently put an intrauterine device (IUD) into his wife's uterus for birth control. I was a little surprised to see her there so early after the insertion. She told me that she really thought the strings were too long and that they should be trimmed. As I started to ask her how she knew that, her husband proceeded to unzip his pants. He had full intentions of pulling his penis out to show me the "red dots" on the head of his penis. I screamed, "Noooooooooooooooo!" This, of course, brought my office staff running into the exam room. It was awkward for all of us with the patient dressed on the exam table and her husband standing with his pants around his ankles. I asked him to please dress. I said, "I promise that I believe you. Now why don't we cut those strings?"

Women sometimes just say funny things in my office. For example, a new patient came in for her annual exam. I thanked her for her trust in coming to me as a physician. She said, "I don't really need much. I am just here for my lube job and transmission check." Another patient told me that she wanted to switch to a female gynecologist. She said, "My last gynecologist did a uterine biopsy on me and told me that I was going to have a little cramp. I realized that he had never had an endometrial biopsy, and he was just whistling up my ass."

Sometimes when someone comes in repeatedly with vaginal infections, I ask them if they have more than one sexual partner. One woman said, "No, but I am a serial monogamist. Is that okay?"

I asked another new patient if she wanted to talk about anything. She thought about it for a minute and said, "I bleed after intercourse, but I think that it is because my husband's fingernails are too long. Can you fix this?" I can't make this up.

I saw a suspicious area on the opening of the vagina in a patient and proceeded to do a biopsy on this spot to make sure that it was not precancerous. She said, "Doctor, I know that you know what you are doing, but please be careful of the button." Don't worry. I would never hurt your button.

A patient had come into the office with suspicions of a urinary tract infection (UTI). We obtained a urine culture and put her on antibiotics. The report revealed that she was on the appropriate antibiotic to treat this particular infection. The bacteria, Escherichia coli (E.coli), which is the most common cause of a UTI, caused the infection. My nurse called her and told her that she had a UTI from the bacteria E.coli. Very quickly she became furious, and my nurse started crying very hard. She came to get me. She told me what had happened, and I got on the phone with the patient. She said, "How dare you accuse me of putting hamburger meat in my vagina!" I explained that E.coli was common bacteria found on the outside of the vagina and was one of the most common causes of urinary tract infections in women. I explained that she was confused with the toxin that E.coli can cause, in some instances, if you eat undercooked meat. She hung up on me.

THE LADY PARTS

24
THE VULVA

"Vulva "is the Latin word for womb or covering. The vulva is what you are looking at when you look between your legs with a mirror. Our outside parts or external genital organs have counterparts in the male external genitals. The vulva consists of several layers that cover and protect the vagina, lubrication glands, the clitoris, and the opening of the tube to the bladder (urethra). There are two sets of "lips" on the external parts of a woman. The outer, fleshy larger lips are called the labia majora. They are also affectionately referred to as the "protectors of the dove" or the mud-flaps. The top and lateral sides of the labia are covered with thick skin, sebaceous (oil-secreting) glands, and hair. The inner sides are smooth and hairless, with some sweat glands. Underneath the skin of the labia majora, there is mostly fat, smooth muscle fibers, nerves, and many blood vessels.

The skin of the labia majora corresponds to the scrotum in the male. In the male the scrotum holds the testicles (gonads) where sperm are created. The female coun-

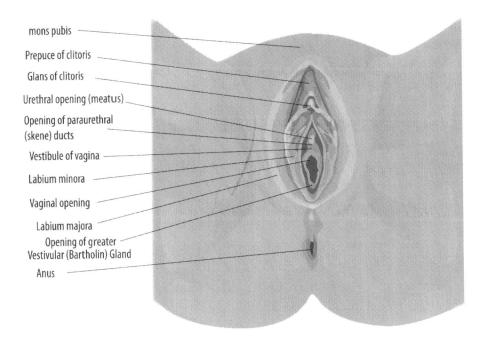

mons pubis

Prepuce of clitoris

Glans of clitoris

Urethral opening (meatus)

Opening of paraurethral
(skene) ducts

Vestibule of vagina

Labium minora

Vaginal opening

Labium majora

Opening of greater
Vestivular (Bartholin) Gland

Anus

terparts to the testicles are the ovaries. As we know, the testicles hurt when they are hit. Our ovaries would hurt if they were hit also, but fortunately they are well protected inside our pelvis. However, sometimes during a pelvic exam an OB/GYN may get a real good grasp of the ovaries between both the internal and external hand and squeeze the ovaries a little. This may make the patient jump a little and cry out; she had her gonads squeezed, and sometimes this is uncomfortable.

The labia majora protect the clitoris, the urethra (the opening of the tube from the bladder), and the opening of the vagina from trauma and potential infections. The thinner, more pigmented, and delicate inner lips (labia minora) join at the top to enclose the clitoris. These small lips join at the top to make the clitoral hood. The clitoral hood and the clitoris have hundreds of nerve endings. The labia majora, labia minora, and clitoris are made up of erectile tissue. Just like the penis, when aroused, a woman's labia majora, labia minora, and the clitoris engorge with blood and become larger. The clitoris is the small, hard bump at the top and between your larger lips. The entire clitoris is actually shaped like the wishbone of a turkey. The only part of the clitoris that you can see is the top of the wishbone where the two sides meet at the top. The clitoris is the female counterpart of the penis, and the only purpose of the clitoris is for sexual arousal. The clitoris differs from a man in that it is much smaller, and it does not have the urethra going through it. However, just like the penis, the clitoris has an erection when stimulated. The arms of the wishbone extend into the body alongside the urethra and the vagina. The parts of the clitoris that become filled with blood during sexual excitement are called the corpora cavernosa and bulbs.

Men and women both know that stimulation of the penis causes a man to have an orgasm. A woman knows that stimulation of the clitoris causes an orgasm. Somewhere along the way, we never told men this important point. If a woman got into bed with her husband with the intention of making love and never touched the penis, never stimulated the penis, and never let the penis touch her, she can be sure that he is not going to have an orgasm. So why do most women accept that their clitoris is not going to be stimulated? This is the number one complaint that I hear from women. They enjoy the closeness that making love brings. They love being held and having their husbands inside them; they love to be kissed, caressed, hugged, and kissed. The same attention is not given to the clitoris that is given to the penis. Never let your partner be ilclitorite.

25
THE VAGINA

In Latin the word vagina means "a sheath for a sword," which is appropriate seeing as the vagina is the canal that accepts the penis. It is the opening between the labia that extend up to the cervix and uterus. The squamous cells of the vagina continually slough off and new ones are made. These cells contain glycogen, which the normal vaginal bacteria ferment to produce lactic acid. This keeps the vagina acidic and inhibits unwanted bacteria that can cause an infection. The vaginal walls are also full of estrogen receptors. When the estrogen receptors are stimulated, the walls of the vagina stay thick and spongy. The more estrogen that is present for the estrogen receptors, the thicker the walls will become and lubrication glands are stimulated to put out mucous. The Bartholin glands are located near the opening of the vagina and secrete a thin, colorless mucous during sexual excitation.

The vagina works kind of like an accordion in that the walls of the vagina have many folds in them, which are called "rugae." When something (a penis or a vibrator or whatever you want) is put into it, it stretches out. The walls of the vagina have two layers of muscle: one running around the vagina and one running along the length of the vagina. The tissue covering the muscles connects with the connective tissue of the bladder, rectum, uterus, and other muscles in the pelvis. When you use muscles to stop the flow of urine or a bowel movement, you are using these muscles. When you have an orgasm, these are the muscles that contract. These muscles can be strengthened by squeezing these muscles many times per day. The working out of these muscles is called Kegel exercises. There are many ways to do Kegel exercises.

26
THE UTERUS AND OVARIES

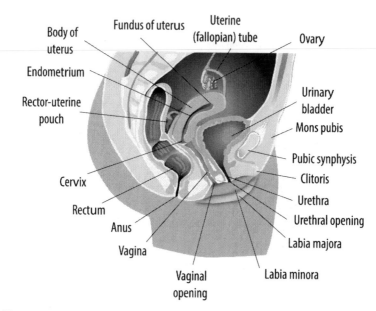

Body of uterus
Fundus of uterus
Uterine (fallopian) tube
Ovary
Endometrium
Rector-uterine pouch
Urinary bladder
Mons pubis
Pubic synphysis
Cervix
Clitoris
Rectum
Urethra
Anus
Urethral opening
Vagina
Labia majora
Vaginal opening
Labia minora

The Uterus

The uterus, more commonly known as the womb, is muscle shaped like a light bulb, or an upside-down pear. Three layers of muscle form the uterus, however, the inside layer is lined with special glandular tissue called the endometrial lining, also known as the endometrium. Menstrual blood forms on this lining. After puberty the estrogen produced by a woman's ovaries stimulates growth of the endometrium. If a woman does not become pregnant, this lining will be expelled about every twenty-eight days. Once menstruation has begun, the size of the uterus is roughly the size of the back of your hand when you make a fist. When the ovaries stop making estrogen in menopause, the uterus usually shrinks to a size that would fit in the palm of a hand. As many women know, the uterus can be a source of unwanted pain and cramping. Women can feel their uterus contracting when they are on their menstrual period. Contractions are muscle cramps, similar to when you get a charley horse in your calf. Sometimes menstrual cramps can cause women to experience a lot of pain, and other times, the pain can be mild.

Occasionally one little muscle cell goes nutty and starts growing and the cells begin multiplying. When this happens, the cells grow enough to make a tumor. The benign muscle tumors that develop are called fibroids. Fibroids are hard, round, masses of muscle cells that can enlarge the uterus. Generally, larger fibroids, and in turn, a larger uterus, will cause heavier menstrual bleeding. About 50 percent of women have fibroids; it is very common. Most fibroids are small and do not cause problems. If you have large fibroids around the time of menopause, your irregular bleeding may be worse than usual.

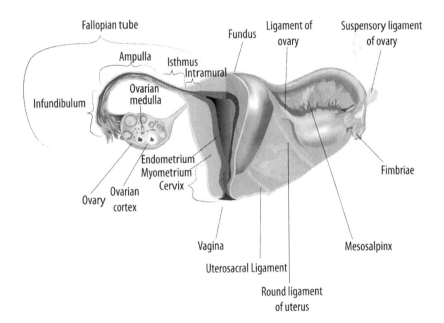

The Ovaries

The ovaries are located next to the uterus and are attached to the uterus by a ligament called the utero-ovarian ligament. In response to signals sent by the brain, the ovaries release a low level of the female hormone estrogen, which gets absorbed into the bloodstream. The estrogen travels to the brain where it bathes the estrogen receptors. When the brain has its receptors full of estrogen, it is happy. From around age eighteen to about forty, the ovaries function beautifully. There may be a "glitch" here or there causing an abnormal menstrual cycle. Nevertheless, for the most part, a perfectly choreographed release of estrogen and progesterone amazingly makes menstrual bleeding regular. Although the following explanation has been simplified, here is how the menstrual cycle works: day one of bleeding = day one of the menstrual cycle. Until I went to medical school, I always thought the first day you bled was the end of your cycle, but it is actually the beginning. At the beginning of the cycle, several eggs are recruited to be "the chosen one."

Several eggs are being recruited

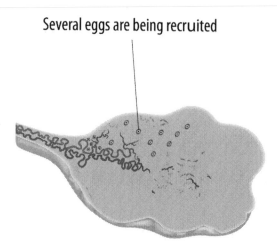

It takes several days for just one egg to be chosen. The egg grows in a fluid-filled cyst called a follicle. If your ovaries are working well, you will make a little cyst on your ovary each month.

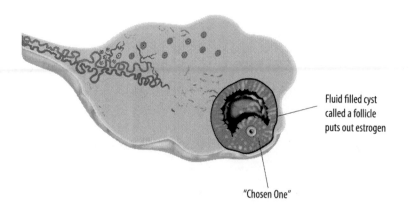

Fluid filled cyst
called a follicle
puts out estrogen

"Chosen One"

The follicle produces the estrogen, and it is released into the blood stream. The estrogen bathes the estrogen receptors in the brain making the brain very happy. The estrogen also makes the menstrual lining form on the uterine walls.

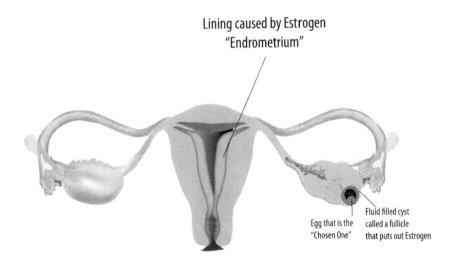

Lining caused by Estrogen
"Endrometrium"

Egg that is the
"Chosen One"

Fluid filled cyst
called a follicle
that puts out Estrogen

Fourteenth day

Around the fourteenth day of the menstrual cycle, a hormone from the brain is released which causes the follicle (or small cyst with an egg in it) to burst, causing ovulation. At this point, the name of the follicle changes to become a corpus luteum. The name is changed because the ruptured cyst now produces progesterone instead of estrogen.

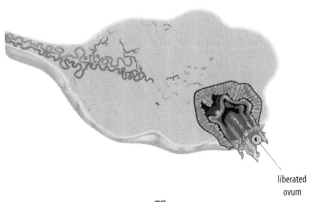

liberated
ovum

The progesterone helps thicken and stabilize the lining in the uterus. If the endometrial lining could be thought of as a type of bed for a potential baby, the progesterone transforms the bed from an old coil spring mattress into a TEMPER-Cloud Luxe mattress.

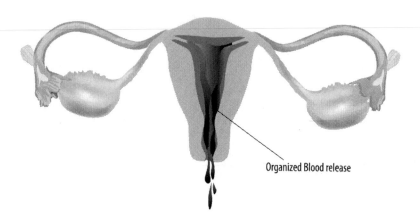

Organized Blood release

The corpus luteum will "die" if there is no fertilization of the egg, which means the progesterone production will stop abruptly. When progesterone is withdrawn, it causes women to release blood from the endometrial cavity.

At this point estrogen levels are very low and the brain's estrogen receptors are without estrogen; the brain is not very happy.

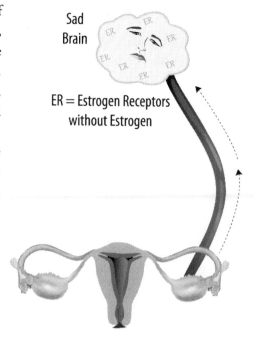

Sad Brain

ER = Estrogen Receptors without Estrogen

The only way for the brain to get estrogen is to make the ovary recruit more follicles, so the brain puts out follicle stimulating hormone (FSH), and new eggs are recruited. The whole process starts over again.

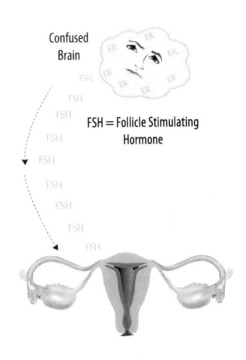

Confused Brain

FSH = Follicle Stimulating Hormone

The perfectly choreographed release of estrogen and progesterone ceases around age forty. Menstrual bleeding becomes irregular and heavy, and ovulation stops being regular.

If there is no ovulation, there is no corpus luteum formed.

If there is no corpus luteum formed, there is no progesterone.

If there is no progesterone, there is no withdrawal of progesterone.

If there is no withdrawal of progesterone, there is no organized release of blood from the uterus.

Any bleeding that does occur is an overgrowth of the endometrial lining. When a woman runs out of eggs completely, there is no way for the brain to stimulate estrogen production.

The brain will keep putting out lots of FSH in an effort to make a follicle. So the higher the FSH levels, the likelihood increases that there are no more eggs available to make a follicle.

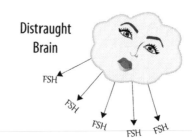

Distraught Brain

FSH = Follicle Stimulating Hormone

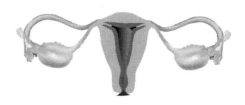

A physician can try to determine whether a woman is menopausal by checking FSH levels. *There is no definitive test for menopause.* Menopause is defined as the absence of menstrual periods for twelve months. It is accompanied by elevated FSH levels. If FSH levels are high, you probably do not have any more eggs and are not having periods. There are no eggs for the FSH to stimulate and your ovaries are destined to shrivel up to almost nothing. Their job is done.

The following is what I tell my patients about FSH levels and what they can expect with regard to their FSH levels and bleeding:

FSH LEVELS	BLEEDING
Less than 20:	You are going to have bleeding
20–40:	Your ovaries are shutting down and you are probably going to have miserable, horrible, heavy periods. Misery bleeding.
40–80:	Who knows what is going to happen? You may have bleeding; you may not.
80–100:	You are probably done.
100 or greater:	You are done.

MENOPAUSE

27
PERIMENOPAUSE

A woman is officially "menopausal" when she has not had a menstrual period for twelve months. However, the "perimenopausal era" is a very ill-defined time frame from about age forty until the time a woman has had no menstrual periods for twelve months. Women have a sense of awareness that they are going through "the change." There are several stages of menopause. The first stage starts around age forty and is caused by poor functioning of the ovaries as the estrogen and progesterone production decreases. This is the reason that women find it difficult to get pregnant after forty years of age. The menstrual cycle stops being regular. Cycles may vary, going from twenty to forty plus days. Instead of a normal menstrual flow, there can be the passage of large blood clots (the feeling that you are laying eggs) and/or unexpected bleeding through clothing.

Emotional changes may occur such as anger, rage, crying, excessive worrying, or anxiety. For this reason, perimenopause is generally not a great time for husbands. Without notice, women in menopause can go from being very pleasant to being cold and hostile. They have been known to go from being extremely peaceful and content to being extremely angry and outraged. Women understand that if they have not had a baby by age forty, the chances of conceiving are low, which can be very distressing. I may have someone in the office say, "Doctor, please hurry up and help me get pregnant! I can hear my eggs cracking."

A patient may have menstrual cycles every couple of months, and they can be intermixed with periods of very heavy bleeding and clotting. Let's face it. The bleeding can be horrendous during perimenopause. I have a great example. When the OB/GYN residents want to schedule someone for a hysterectomy, I want to make sure that this degree of intervention is indicated. Most of the time we do not schedule anyone for a hysterectomy for heavy bleeding unless they have tried conservative methods first. These methods may be birth control pills, a progesterone intrauterine device (IUD), or an endometrial ablation. Occasionally we bypass these conservative methods if the patient has a situation that does not apply here. For example, if a patient's abnormal bleeding is caused by large uterine fibroids (benign uterine tumors), conservative methods of treatment may not work. The residents came into my office and informed me that they had a good candidate for a hysterectomy for heavy bleeding and clotting. I asked if the patient had tried any conservative methods to control the bleeding. The residents said that she had not tried anything conservative. Her story, however, was so good that they felt she should bypass conservative methods in this situation. I rolled my eyes and said that she had really better have a good story in order to bypass the usual order of treatment. The resident felt I should hear the story from the patient personally. I agreed. I went into the examination room and introduced myself as the Attending Physician.

The patient stated that she needed a hysterectomy as soon as possible. I asked why she felt so strongly about needing such a major surgery. She looked at me very calmly and said, "Because, I never want to give another blow job." What? I sat down. She said, "Doctor, I bleed so much that I soak the sheets at night. I bleed through my clothes during the day. I bleed so much that my husband will not have sex with me anymore; he feels uncomfortable with all the blood. Therefore, I have to give him blowjobs. I hate blowjobs. I never want to give another blowjob. Please help me."

I said, "I have operating room time on Tuesdays. How soon would you like your hysterectomy?"

She said, "Tuesday."

I said, "Done."

The second stage of menopause starts in the mid-forties. It results in even less ovarian estrogen function and a complete disruption of the estrogen and progesterone environment. A patient may have menstrual cycles every couple of months, and they can be intermixed with periods of very heavy bleeding and clotting. This is when hot flashes may start. Usually they start at night (night flushes), and may cause you to wake up soaked and hot. Then you may promptly become freezing cold. The hot flashes may start happening during the day, and your scalp and head drip sweat at the most inopportune times. Actually, I think that there is a force, which is pushing hot water up to your neck, face, and eventually your scalp. This pressure pushes the water out of each hair follicle simultaneously as the water then drips off of the end of enough hair that you look like you have run a mile or two, but not enough that you just got out of the shower. You feel as if you just left the gym and need a shower. Unfortunately, this occurs most often while you are doing something important. This stage ends twelve months after the last menstrual period. Now you enter the last stage at which time you are officially menopausal. Women will come in and tell me that their ovaries are sputtering.

"Doctor, I hate having my period; when do I get to the pause part?"

"Doctor, I am sweating like a slut! Help me!"

"I have been waiting so long for menopause; it is like being in a bad marriage and waiting for a divorce!"

Women are so funny during this time of life. When you get too tired of crying, you just have to laugh. I had given one of my patients the diagnosis of lichen sclerosis, which is a skin condition that postmenopausal women get. It makes the outside of the vagina (and the whole area) itch terribly, scar, and turn white. When I came in the room she said, "Remember me? I am the patient that has moss growing on the north side of my bush!"

Another patient said, "I told my husband that I don't like myself today, so you can imagine where you stand."

"I have entered the snapdragon part of my life; part of me has snapped and the rest of me is draggin'."

This is a bad time for intimate partners. One patient told me that she and her husband were going through changes at the same time. "He is going through Man-o-Pause while I am going through menopause; we hate each other."

"My husband thinks that I have hearing problems and wants me to talk to you about it. Actually, nothing is wrong with my hearing. I just choose to ignore him and let him think that I cannot hear him. I am telling you this so that I can tell him that I talked to you about it."

A woman came in and told me that the bruises on her arms and legs were from her husband. She said, "He kept hitting me, so I shot and killed him. He is home dead in our bathroom." Horrified, scared, and shocked, I said, "Oh my God, really?" She said, "No, but I wish that I was telling a true story. I think that I need help."

I walked in on a patient crying in my exam room. She said, "I am so emotional! I came home crying the other day, and my husband thought that I was just happy to see him. We been married long enough that he should know better than that."

"Doctor, I have issues with my tissues."

"Doctor, I think that I am spasmatic." I said, "Do you mean asthmatic?" She said, "No, spasmatic. I spaz out all the time."

"You have to help me, I have Prozac poop out."

I asked one patient if I could do a rectal exam on her. She said, "Sure, I never want anything done to me that is half-ass." Funny.

85

28
Y-T-R-E-B-U-P

When I try to explain the trials and tribulations of menopause to my patients, I try to relate it to another horrible time of our lives, puberty. If you think about it, menopause is puberty in reverse. When we are about eight years old, our hormones start pumping out, but we do not really look any different until we are about twelve years old, that is, start getting boobies and pubic hair. Well, even though we get our first menstrual period at around thirteen or fourteen years of age, puberty is not finished until around eighteen, when the breasts are fully developed and the hips complete their curvature. It takes about ten years for the entire pubertal process to complete. Then, we have about twenty years of relative stability; our periods are regular, it is not difficult to get pregnant (for most women), and our periods are pretty much uniform in terms of time in between them and the amount of days we bleed. Then at around thirty-eight years of age, our ovaries start to fail. Our periods start to stay on longer and get closer together or farther apart. For most women it is very difficult to get pregnant after the age of thirty-five.

Now, let us go back to puberty. How do we describe puberty in our teenagers? They are moody. They cry hysterically one minute; they are happy the next. They cannot control their emotions. They slam doors, call their parents stupid, and tell them that they hate them; then they come down and cry and tell you they are sorry. I remember driving my daughter home from school last year (she was fifteen), and she was telling me about something funny that happened with her friends. She was laughing hysterically. It was great. I was laughing hysterically also, even though I could hardly understand what she was saying. It was one of those moments that I will remember my whole life. My beautiful daughter and I were laughing hysterically and trying not to pee in our pants. We lived on Tybee Island, and at that moment we were driving past miles of the most beautiful marshes, rivers, and shrimp boats that you could ever envision. I gently closed my eyes to thank God for everything—the moment with my daughter that I would always remember, the beautiful place where I lived, the peacefulness of the day, and for all the things for which I had to be thankful. Well, this moment of thanks with God was interrupted by the most sorrowful, loud, heartbreaking sobbing, wailing, and crying that you could ever imagine. I almost screamed when I heard her cry, because it frightened me. What happened? She proceeded to try to tell me that there were some people at school that were making fun of her, and she never wanted to go to school again as long as she lived. She cried for two hours. I tried to console her when we got home, but I just did not understand. I tried to hold her, but I was making her hot. I gave her head a million kisses and told her that I loved her, but I was ruining her hair. She said, "You just don't understand because things are so much more complicated in my generation." She wanted to be left alone. Later that night, she came up to the kitchen to get some milk, and I asked her if she was okay. She said, in a completely normal voice, "Yeah, why?"

Lord, please give me patience. I just lost six months off my life worrying about her, and she does not even remember why or even that she was crying. Sound familiar? When our ovaries fail, I think that we go through all the emotions of puberty in reverse. To make matters worse, it takes longer to complete the process. It takes about ten years for your ovaries to work well, but it takes about fifteen years for them to fail. Not only do the emotions of puberty happen again in menopause, but everything else does too. The acne returns. Really.

I have more women who take Accutane (a drug for acne) in their forties than I do in their teens. How unfair is that? In addition, the weight gain is very unfair. When I give lectures on puberty to fourth and fifth grade girls, I always talk to them about the weight gain of puberty. I tell them that they and their girlfriends will put on some weight around the time (before and after) they get their first period. It is completely unfair that they will put on weight before they have their growth spurt and get taller. Unfortunately, they may get a little chubby for a while. I tell them that this is normal and it is going to be okay; they are all going to get their growth spurt and the weight should even out eventually. Someday they too will look like the high school girls of which they are so jealous. I also point out that the boys are the lucky ones. They get tall before they put on weight. They get tall and weirdly skinny and lanky before they put on weight and look more like young men. In menopause we start out looking good, and then we put on weight. The problem is that we never get out of that stage. It would be fine if our bodies looked like small, lanky prepubescent girls, but we are stuck in that miserable weight gain stage. We never get out. It is also a cruel twist of fate to go through menopause when your child is going through puberty.

29
TREATING THE BLEEDING

The bleeding abnormalities in menopause can be horrible. Bleeding during this time of your life must be considered a "sign" of something bad going on and treated as such. The number one thing your doctor must do is make sure you do not have cancer in your vagina, bladder, urinary tract, cervix, uterus, fallopian tubes, or ovaries. After that determination has been made, there are many options to consider. One option for treating the bleeding is taking oral contraceptive pills (OCPs or birth control pills). Many women take pills and do very well. A woman who takes birth control pills tends not to have abnormal bleeding. I have moved away from starting patients on birth control pills because I have had so much success with the Mirena IUD. Not only is an IUD less expensive in the long run, the risk factor for blood clots and strokes are lower than with OCPs. It is comforting to know that the Mirena IUD does not increase risk of stroke.

A second option for treating (or stopping) abnormal bleeding is a minor surgical procedure called endometrial ablation. This is not my first choice because it involves surgery, and for me, I feel like I am taking better care of you if I keep out of the operating room. There are many physicians who are set up to do endometrial ablations in their offices. Endometrial ablation is a procedure that destroys (ablates) the endometrial lining and works wonderfully in this age group. The endometrium is burned off, and the endometrial cavity scars down, which usually reduces or prevents uterine bleeding. OB/GYNs use this surgery frequently in women who do not wish to use any hormones (progesterone IUD or birth control pills), do not get better on the hormonal options, and do not desire to have any more children.

The destruction of the inside lining of the uterus can be performed in several different ways. All the different techniques are used frequently by OB/GYNs. You can burn the uterine lining directly with a bipolar radio-frequency cauterization device called Novasure. This device is put into the uterine cavity (where the baby would be if you were pregnant) and opened up in a triangular fashion. The endometrial cavity is then burned. Another way to destroy the endometrium is to put very hot water directly into the uterus. The water is circulated throughout the cavity. This is called Hydro-Therm-Ablator (HTA for short). We can also put the hot water into the uterus confined inside a balloon. This is called Thermachoice. We can use microwaves to burn the cavity, Microwave Endometrial Ablation, or we can freeze the inner lining with a device called Her Option. If you look up endometrial ablation, you will find various statistics describing the rate of amenorrhea (lack of bleeding). In my experience, I find that fifty percent of women have no more bleeding and are profoundly happy. They are put to sleep, and when they wake up, they have no more periods. When they come in for their annual exams, they think that you hung the moon. They send their friends to come in to see you. Twenty-five percent of patients have much lighter periods. They wish that they were in the fifty percent that have no periods, but still, their lives are so much better. I wish they had no periods also, but I am happy that that they are better. This procedure does not really help about 25 percent of patients. This is profoundly disappointing to the patient and the physician. Here, the physician has taken someone to the operating room and she is no better off than before she went in. I always prepare my patients for this outcome. I am probably overestimating, because I only remember the patients in which the procedure did not work. You generally do not remember all the happy people; a physician remembers the people who are disappointed. Then there are some women in the first two groups who start bleeding terribly again. Just shoot me.

Sometimes the bleeding starts up again after a couple of years. The body has a unique ability to heal itself. The treated areas heal or maybe the destruction did not go deep enough. It does not really matter why it happened; they are bleeding again. No physician likes having a disappointed patient. I really have better luck stopping bleeding with the progesterone IUD. I prefer to go from less invasive procedures and move toward more invasive procedures. I would rather someone try the IUD first. If it did not work well, they could always do an ablation. You cannot rely on doing the ablation first and then putting in the progesterone IUD. The cavity becomes so scarred down that the IUD cannot get in there. There are some reports of OB/GYNs putting in the IUD right after an ablation (while they are still in the operating room); however, there is not much data on this. Again, this is something that must be individualized to each specific patient. There is no right answer. When researchers and statisticians look at lots of studies to see how women fared long-term after an ablation, the analyses show that around 20-25 percent of women had to have additional surgery for abnormal bleeding. It has nothing to do with the type of ablation that is performed or the experience level of the surgeon. In most cases they will have another ablation or a hysterectomy. To do an ablation, I really prefer you to be older than forty years of age. The older you are, the less likely that you will start bleeding again. Remember, your body is going to decrease the blood supply to the uterine lining when you go through menopause. Obviously, you need to have completed your family when you do an ablation. It is a bit dangerous to get pregnant after an ablation because the baby's placenta may not be able to get the blood supply it needs for the baby to grow. There is a very high chance of preterm delivery of the baby before it can live on its own. If the pregnancy does make it into the last trimester, it may be difficult to get the placenta off the uterus after the baby is born, which results in a significant blood loss in the mother. When I do an endometrial ablation, I also do a tubal ligation at the same time so that I do not have to worry about those complications. Some women come in and just want a hysterectomy. They just want it out. I am sure that you can always find an OB/GYN to do this. This would be appropriate if you had a big uterus full of benign fibroid tumors, but if you are having miserable peri-menopausal bleeding, you should go through the conservative treatment first: OCPs, Mirena IUD, or ablation. A hysterectomy is major surgery. Bad things can go wrong during any surgery but are more likely to go wrong if it is a major surgery. If I take you to the operating room to do major surgery and something goes wrong such as a bowel injury, terrible blood loss, or God forbid, death, I will have to live with the fact that I did not do something conservative first.

30
PROGESTERONE IUDS

After making sure that my patients have no pre-cancer or cancer in their genital organs, I recommend they treat this miserable time of mood swings, exacerbated PMS, and heavy irregular bleeding by using a progesterone-coated intrauterine device. Many of you are thinking to yourself, "I can't get pregnant now anyway, and IUDs are very dangerous!"

IUD. Three little letters which can terrify women if mentioned in an OB/GYN's office. Those of us that are a little older remember friends, acquaintances, and unfortunate women that we read about in women's magazines who had terrible complications from an IUD (intrauterine device). In the 1960's and 1970's, there absolutely was a problem with a particular IUD, the Dalkon Shield. This IUD gave all of them a bad name. The Dalkon Shield had several flaws in it that tremendously increased the risk of severe pelvic infection. Once this was understood, the Dalkon Shield was taken off the market. Unfortunately, the use of this form of contraception all but stopped. Actually, intrauterine contraception is one of the safest and most effective methods of contraception available today.

Since the 1970's there has only been one copper-releasing IUD on the market which is called the Paragard IUD. In 2002 only 2 percent of contraceptive users in the United States chose to use IUDs; this number increased to 8 percent by 2009. Because of legal battles and bad press that occurred in the 1970's, the United States lags far behind other countries in terms of IUD use. For comparison, IUDs are used by over 50 percent of women using contraception in Asia and almost thirty percent of female contraceptive users in Europe. Around 1990, a progesterone-releasing IUD came on the market in the United States. The brand name of this product is called Mirena. If you are a female and hate your periods as much as I do, you need to know about the Mirena IUD. If you are a perimenopausal female between the ages of forty and fifty-five years and are horrified to find that almost overnight your periods changed, or if your menstrual periods went from annoying and tolerable to a bloodletting event comparable to hanging a pig upside down by its feet and slitting its throat, then you need to know about the Mirena IUD.

This T-shaped IUD is coated in a small amount (52 milligrams) of a very common progesterone (levonorgestrel) that is found in some birth-control pills. The Mirena IUD releases minute amounts (20 micrograms) locally into the uterine cavity each day. This is much less progesterone than is found in progesterone implants or progesterone only birth-control pills. The Mirena IUD does not affect the ovary's production of estrogen and does not contain any estrogen at all. Fortunately, the major side effect is that most women have very light or no menstrual periods.

When I stopped delivering precious little babies in 2006, my patient base went from being a majority of women twenty to forty years of age to a majority being forty to sixty years of age. The number one complaint in women this age is heavy perimenopausal bleeding. Needless to say, the Mirena IUD is my number one recommendation to treat this type of bleeding. After this IUD is placed, most women have three to six months of nuisance bleeding. Most of my patients do not need it for birth control because they have already had their fallopian tubes tied or their partner has had a vasectomy. These patients use it to reduce heavy menstrual bleeding, severe pain with periods, or for premenstrual syndrome (PMS). The package insert says that women should not use the Mirena IUD if they are bothered by *not* having a period.

The company has recently produced another progesterone-releasing IUD that has less progesterone in it, Skyla IUD. Skyla users usually have a light period, whereas Mirena users usually do not have periods. Some women are comforted by the presence of their menses each month, and if that is you, Skyla would be a better option. The Skyla IUD was made a bit smaller to be used in younger women. The Skyla IUD can be used in any young girl that would like long-term birth control and can tolerate the insertion procedure. I do what is called a para-cervical block using a local anesthetic on all my patients that receive an IUD. It is the injection of local anesthesia into the cervix to give them relief of pain. The IUD takes about ten seconds to put into the uterine cavity.

The Mirena IUD is used by many OB/GYNs as an alternative to oral progesterone in patients that want estrogen therapy. This use for the Mirena IUD is common, but it is off-label; this means that it is not approved by the FDA specifically for this use.

The Mirena IUD may decrease pain from endometriosis, delay recurrence of endometriosis after surgery, and can be used in women who are on blood thinners. Many women on blood thinners such as warfarin (Coumadin) have heavy menstrual bleeding. These patients usually come in and want a hysterectomy because they are tired of the heavy bleeding. As you can imagine, these patients are at a very high risk for surgery because of their use of blood thinners. A Mirena IUD is a perfect option and keeps them out of surgery. What can I say that is bad about Mirena IUD? Some women continue to bleed irregularly after the first three to six months and are just tired of it. Women do not enjoy the "unscheduled" bleeding that can occur with this product. There are women who develop acne, breast tenderness, and/or mood swings. However, I find that these symptoms usually subside if they give it a few more months. You may have guessed by now that I use this product. Actually, besides having my children and getting married, this is the best thing that I have done for myself in my life. I do not have financial affiliation with this company (Bayer Pharmaceuticals).

31
MENOPAUSE

The third stage of menopause is when you are completely menopausal. You are completely menopausal, and it is official when a woman has no periods (amenorrhea) for a full year, you have no more eggs in the ovaries, and your ovaries do not make any more estrogen.

The real definition (according to Dr. Pam) is: After an internal light switch goes off that is triggered by the lack of estrogen, the ovaries squinch up, scream, and stop working. This causes the estrogen receptors in the brain (which now have no estrogen) to also scream, causing general tearfulness, memory loss, significant and profound weight gain (no matter how little you eat), emotional lability, and intermittent, internal rage interfaced with profound sadness and sympathy leading to an inability to watch chick flicks, romantic comedies, Lifetime Television, Hallmark commercials, or any program that deals with children or animals without bursting into tears. Any thoughts of sexual intercourse are profoundly suppressed and eventually disappear completely. Road rage increases rapidly and frequently, and correlates exactly to how much your husband and/or children made you angry last night (right before you started crying). One patient reported, "My whole life is Murphy's Law." Everything is going so wrong lately that I think that I have been sleeping with Murphy. Recently things have been so bad; I think that I have been giving him a blowjob." Another patient called and said, "My husband and I have had a budgetary stricture, and we lost our insurance." She could not afford to come in. She asked, "Can I get a refill on my hormones? If not, will you testify at his murder trial?"

Unfortunately, everything that we have is affected by gravity after menopause. The fat on our arms hangs down, your stomach folds over your pants, your breasts go south, and your bladder falls out. One woman said to me, "Doctor, you know how men have testicles?" Yes. "Well, my breasts hang down so low now that I call them breasticles." Another patient informed me that it was not going to be long before she could tell the temperature of the floor just by taking off her bra. "Well, at the rate my breasts are falling, my nipples will touch the floor soon." One woman informed me that she was tired of having surgery because everything was falling down. When I told her that her bladder was falling she said, "I am just going to duct tape my bladder to my leg."

I often tell the following joke in the office when women complain about their breasts falling down. An older woman's husband died after sixty-five years of marriage. She missed him terribly and wanted to join him in heaven. She went out and bought a gun and some bullets. She was not completely sure exactly where her heart was so she called her doctor to ask him. He said, "Your heart is just below your left nipple." She thanked him and said good-bye. She was admitted to the hospital that evening with a gunshot wound to her left knee.

Weight Gain

The weight gain in menopause is serious. There is no way that so many women can come into the office complaining of the same thing. There would have to be some type of mass hysteria or something. When a woman gains weight, it affects her whole life. It is not just from the standpoint of how she looks for her husband, but how she feels about herself. If she does not want to look at herself naked, there is a very good chance that her husband is not going to see her naked either. Women come in frantic about their weight. I know that they are telling the truth when they come in saying that they are barely eating anything and keep gaining. The key to surviving the weight gain of menopause is a regimented exercise program. The most frequent response that I hear when I ask if my patient is exercising regularly is that she exercises while she is working. So many patients feel that when they are running around at work and on their feet all day they are getting adequate exercise. I want so much to tell them that this is appropriate exercise; unfortunately it does not even come close. In order to counteract whatever it is that makes us gain weight around the perimenopause, we must have a regimented exercise program. There must be time specifically set aside for exercise. The minimum time is thirty minutes per day for at least three days a week. I really do not think that this is enough. The women who do the best with weight management are those that exercise six to seven days per week.

Something happens at this point in our lives, and we have to work out like dogs. I hate it; it sounds very cruel. I am so very sorry, but you must have a specific, structured, stand-alone exercise program. I know that you do not have time to do it, but you have to make the time. Just as you have to give yourself forty-five min-utes in the morning to get ready, you have to make this a necessary part of your day. Take it one day at a time. If you do not make exercise part of your daily regimen, the weight will get away from you. The weight gain is, in my opinion, directly related to the lack of libido. Again, if you do not like the way you look naked, there is a good chance that your husband is not going to see you naked ei-ther.

Low Libido

The lack of libido is as significant as the weight gain. Some physicians give their female patients Viagra and say that their patients do very well with it. I have tried giving it to many patients. I have not had the results that they have had; I have not had one patient ask me for a refill. Interestingly, not one patient has ever asked me for a refill of Viagra for their husband.

Hmmmm . . .

32
MEMORY LOSS

I'm sorry. I can't remember what I was going to say about that. It is not funny; it is actually frightening. Menopausal patients routinely come into my office, lean forward, and whisper, even though I am the only person who can hear them, "I think I have Alzheimer's disease." I know what you mean.

My children can text me five times that we need milk and bread; they text me so much that I get aggravated with them. But, I forget the milk. Even worse, I pass a grocery store on the way home. One time, after a long day and multiple texts to pick up milk, I passed the grocery store, said a little prayer of thanks that I did not have to go in, and went home. Another time, the kids were in the bed with me because my husband was out of town. It was family movie night. I locked up the house, came back in the bedroom, and told them that I was putting on the house alarm. I told them not to open any doors or windows. Then I walked to the door in my bedroom and opened the door for the dog to go out. As the alarm was screaming, my daughter said, "Mom, you are scaring me." My son said, "Mom, are you kidding us?" I said, "Yes." No. Oh my God! Did I really just do that? I once was at the office and forgot to go get my children at school when they were about five years old. The police called me because it was getting dark, and they were worried about them. You should all be feeling better now about yourselves. Do we have dementia?

Dementia is a decrease in mental function that involves learning and memory, language, function, attention, motor skills, and social memory. We all can relate to social memory. Let me give you an example, which will make you feel great about not remembering anyone's name. I was in church one Sunday morning, and two of my son's best friends had spent the night and came to church with us. At the end of each service, we ask visitors to stand and introduce themselves, and the congregation welcomes them. Well, I stood up to introduce these two boys that I love as much as my own children. I stood up to introduce these two boys that have stayed in my home overnight no less than a hundred times over ten years. I stood up to introduce these two boys that I would protect with my life as much as I would protect my own children. I stood up, had them stand up, and then could not remember their names. The whole church looked at me as though I were crazy. The boys looked at me as if I was crazy. My children and husband looked at me as if I was crazy. I said, "I'm sorry, I just had a menopausal moment." The women laughed, and the men just nodded. My children are still amazed. Even after I sat down, it took me thirty seconds to remember their names. Humiliating. To get the diagnosis of dementia, the memory loss has to be severe enough to interfere with daily function and independence. So please start feeling better about yourself. Alzheimer's disease is the most common form of dementia in the elderly and accounts for up to eighty percent of cases. We all realize this, because we all know someone who is affected by Alzheimer's. It should also make you feel better to know that most people with dementia are brought to their physician by their family. Self-reported memory loss does not appear to correlate with the development of dementia. Informant-reported memory loss in which a family member reports the memory loss to the physician is a better predictor of the presence and future development of dementia. Patients that have dementia have trouble retaining new information, handling complex tasks, such as balancing a checkbook, reasoning, and getting lost in familiar places. You do not get lost in the mall or your favorite boutique. You may not remember why you walked into a room fifty-six times today, but you remember where your hair salon is located. In fact you can probably give me exact directions from where you are located right now.

A Mini-Mental State Examination (MMSE) is the most widely used test for dementia in U.S. clinical practice. Have someone give you the following test. You will feel better about your memory loss almost immediately. If you do not, you need to get your family to take you to your physician.

Mini-Mental State Examination

5 pts.	What is the complete date and season? (time, day, month, year, season)
5 pts.	Where are you exactly? (1 pt. each; country, state, county, town, address)
1 pt.	Name three objects. (Patient repeats the name of all three objects after hearing them said aloud)
5 pts.	Count backwards from 100 by sevens (stop after five answers)
OR	
1 pt. each	Spell WORLD backwards
1 pt. each	Ask the patient to repeat the three objects you mentioned earlier
1 pt. each	Show the patient a pencil and a wristwatch. Ask them to name the objects.
1 pt.	Ask the patient to repeat the sentence: "No ifs, ands, or buts."

(One chance)

1 pt. each   Follow a three-stage command: "Take a paper in your right hand, fold it in half, and put it on the floor."

1 pt.   On a blank piece of paper write: "Close your eyes." Ask the patient to read it and do what it says.

1 pt.   Give the patient a blank piece of paper. Ask them to write any sentence. (The sentence must contain a noun and verb and be sensible.)

1 pt.   Ask the patient to copy a design (e.g. two intersecting pentagons; all 10 angles must be present and two must intersect)

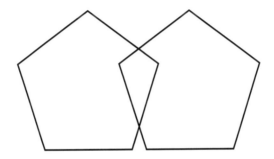

Maximum score: 30 points

A score less than twenty-four is suggestive of dementia. I make a point to tell my patients that if they had the type of memory loss that they should be worried about, they probably would not know they had it. I think people are so overloaded with daily tasks and information that our brains (hard drives) become too full. I tell my kids that I have to forget (delete) something before I can remember (upload) something new. My husband and I have recently started watching "Brain Games" on the National Geographic Channel. Another option for scientific brain training is www.lumosity.com. The idea is to keep your brain working.

33
TAKE THE CAST OFF YOUR VAGINA

One of the best therapies for menopause is exercise. I have many patients who feel that their lives have been changed by doing yoga and Pilates. Many of the health food stores have herbal remedies for the symptoms of menopause. If these work for you, no one will be happier for you than me. I wish every woman could get through menopause without taking hormones. The side effects frighten me also; unfortunately nothing works as well as estrogen replacement therapy. Many women stop taking their hormone replacement therapy and go a bit "bonkers." Many call or come back in the office to renew their prescription.

One woman told me, "I stopped my estrogen because of my fear of cancer. But, I am chewing on all the doorknobs in the house, so I think I should get my prescription renewed." Another patient came in and told me that she lost herself when she went off her hormones. She said, "I know that I'm in there somewhere, I just can't find myself." Another patient came in and said, "I am just a big bag of daddy issues and anger!" Over the next thirty years, probably fifty million women are going to reach menopause. The life expectancy for women is around eighty-five years of age now. What does that mean to me as a gynecologist? It means that I have to keep your vagina working for thirty-five years after menopause (the average age of menopause being fifty-one). You may read this statement and think that I am out of my mind. If you are in your forties and still have children at home, you are probably not having sex that much now. You may think that you cannot wait until menopause, thinking that you do not have to do it anymore. You may have heard that once men start taking medication for hypertension or diabetes, they will not be able to have an erection any longer.

Well, ladies, the fact of the matter is that we are in the Viagra generation. The usual scenario is this: Around fifty to sixty years of age, men are frequently put on medications that can affect their ability to have an erection. Also, the medical problem causes the problem with erections. High cholesterol, high blood pressure, and diabetes cause damage to the little vessels in the body. The vessels that are the farthest away from the heart are smaller and more affected. That is why diabetics have the most problems with their feet. There are many little vessels in the penis. The blood just cannot get in there to maintain an erection. Now, there is a lot of snuggling going on at home and in the bedroom. There is also attention, the kind that we like, that is talking. We women are happy to just snuggle for the rest of our lives. The problem is that without use, your vagina is going to shrivel up. Let me give you an example that I tell my patients. Most moms have had the unfortunate experience of having their child break a bone. It is scary at first and surgery may be needed. However, after that, everyone resigns himself or herself that you just have to put up with a cast for six to twelve weeks while it heals. They get all their friends to write on it and take advantage of the "I can't do any chores" part of their incapacitation.

If you have ever been present when the cast comes off, you know that event is almost as nasty as the break itself (without the pain). The smell is terrible from the arm or leg not being washed and aired out; but worse, the arm looks horrible. The skin is white and the muscles are limp and hanging. This is because the brain has decreased the blood supply to this part of body. It has not been used, the muscles are atrophic (limp and thin), the blood vessels close to the surface are not being used much, and the arm looks a little dead. Now, as soon as the kid starts using it again and running around and playing, the muscles and blood supply gear back up. In a few weeks the arm is looking normal again. Another analogy is frostbite. If someone is stuck out in the cold for extended periods, then the brain is going to divert the blood supply to protect the major organs. The blood supply to the brain, heart, liver, kidneys, pancreas, spleen, and intestines is going to be protected with the warm blood while the fingers and hands, toes and feet, and nose and ears are left to fend for themselves. These areas get frostbite first because the blood supply is intentionally diverted away from nonessential parts to preserve your life. You must think of the vagina as an organ. If you do not use it, it is going to lose its blood supply, thin out, and turn white. The thickness of the mucosa (the skin of the vaginal wall) is going to decrease. The lubrication glands are going to stop producing mucous, and the tissue is going to become very dry. You must keep up the use of your vagina thereby keeping up the blood supply, or it is going to dry up. The vagina will decrease in diameter and will decrease in length.

So, let us go back to the house and the bedroom. While you are happy in the no-intercourse, "snuggly" part of your marriage, I promise you that your husband has never gone twenty-four hours without thinking about having sex again. In my experience it takes men three to five years to get the guts up to see a doctor that will prescribe Viagra. I also promise you that the day that they come home with that little blue pill, their penis will work. It will work well. It will work much better than it did before the diabetes and hypertension. It will work not only the day that they bring the Viagra home, but it will work thirty minutes after they take it. To make it worse, and to a lot of older women's utter horror, it sometimes works a couple of times in one night.

Therefore, after three to five years of a little snuggling and lots of talking, you have to have intercourse, a lot. Even in women who enjoyed intercourse tremendously in their younger years there is considerable pain now during penetration. It makes sense, right? You have had a cast on your vagina for three to five years. Your next phone call is to your gynecologist. You are going to get an appointment and ask him or her to fix this. It is just not that easy. It took five years to get in this terrible, bloodless, dry shape; it may take you several years to get it back. It is not just the lack of use; it is also menopause. Remember, menopause is the complete cessation of menstrual periods for a period of one year. That means that you have no more eggs in your ovaries, which means that you have no more estrogen being produced by them. All the tissue in your vagina and those surrounding areas has estrogen receptors. If these receptors have estrogen to bind to them, they will keep working. After menopause the estrogen receptors are not bound to estrogen, and they "shut off." In a roundabout way these receptors are the on/off button for your vagina, not to be confused with the on button that helps you have the orgasm (your clitoris).

Unfortunately, there is another way that the blood supply to the vagina is shut off by your body. Almost half of the blood supply to the vagina comes from the uterus. After menopause, that is after there are no more periods, the body does not need the uterus or ovaries anymore. The brain "knows" this and has already decreased the blood supply to the uterus and ovaries. The uterus and ovaries shrink up to almost nothing. A normal size uterus in a menstruating woman is about the size of your fist. A few years after menopause, it can fit in the palm of your hand and not even touch your fingers. The ovaries shrink up as well. I recently did a hysterectomy on a fifty-nine-year-old woman because her uterus was falling out. My patient wanted a picture of her uterus and ovaries. To give an idea of to what extent her ovaries shrunk up, I put my pinky fingernail next to her ovary. They were about the same size. She said, "That's it?" Yep, those bad boys were not hurting y in there.

34
PROTECT YOUR VAGINA

The best thing that you can do is keep her in shape. When I encounter a woman who is in the second stage of perimenopause (very heavy periods that are spacing out and hot flashes are present), I talk to them about protecting their vaginas from atrophy (shrinking and drying up). The vaginal symptoms of vaginal atrophy are dryness, burning, itching, pain with intercourse, non-odiferous vaginal discharge, bleeding from the walls of the vagina, and bleeding from the opening of the vagina. There are also symptoms of the urinary tract (the bladder and the tube from the bladder to the outside) that are caused by the lack of estrogen. The skin (mucosa) of the urethra (the tube from the bladder to the outside) also gets thin and results in pain with urination, burning with urination, and, in severe cases, bleeding from the outside of the urethra. Women also get an increase in the number of urinary tract infections. The urethra loses the thickness around the opening, which helps keep out bacteria. As an aside, if a woman is having bleeding from the vagina, cervix, or from the urinary tract, she must be evaluated first for cancer. The bleeding from the uterus could be uterine or cervical cancer, and the bleeding from the tube coming from the bladder can be kidney, bladder, or urethral cancer. Once this is ruled out, and all infectious causes of the bleeding are treated, the patient can be treated for her lack of estrogen. Other names for vaginal atrophy are vulvovaginal atrophy, urogenital atrophy, and atrophic vaginitis. Women who have this problem may not be "officially menopausal." For example, women who are being treated for breast cancer get placed on anti-estrogen drugs. If she is premenopausal, she may be put on Tamoxifen, which is an oral chemotherapy (anti-estrogen drug) for breast cancer. If she is postmenopausal, she may be put on a drug called an aromatase inhibitor. These drugs are used in breast cancer treatment to stop the production of estrogen. Aromatase inhibitors work by blocking the enzyme aromatase, which turns the other hormones, such as the male hormone, "testosterone," into small amounts of estrogen in the body. If you take this, less estrogen is available to stimulate the growth of potential breast cancer cells. Aromatase inhibitors cannot stop the ovaries from making estrogen, so aromatase inhibitors only work in postmenopausal women. There are three different aromatase inhibitors: Arimidex (anastrozole), Aromasin (exemestane), and Femara (letrozole).

These drugs will cause terrible vaginal dryness because they stop production of estrogen.

Consider a woman breast-feeding. In this situation, she is in a very low-estrogen state. The ovaries are not working well to pass out an egg because of the hormone produced in the brain (prolactin) that helps create breast milk. Please do not use breast-feeding for birth control. The ovaries have a unique ability to work when they are not supposed to, just ask any obstetrician. These women may have very significant symptoms of vaginal burning and dryness. The best way to keep it in shape is to use it. Use it every day if possible. I know that you do not have the time, and more specifically, you do not have the need for intercourse every day. This is unrealistic. Of course, you may have a Y chromosome, and this is not such a far-fetched or terrible idea. Therefore, really, for women, this is at the bottom of the list. Women who are sexually active with a partner or through masturbation (a vibrator is especially effective) have fewer symptoms related to vaginal atrophy.

THE "E" WORD: ESTROGEN

35
VAGINAL ESTROGEN

The best thing to prevent vaginal atrophy after menopause is vaginal estrogen placement. There are three ways to give local estrogen to all of those receptors in and around your vagina and bladder: Vaginal estrogen cream, a vaginal estrogen pill, and a vaginal estrogen ring.

The first option is the vaginal cream. It works very well. There are two FDA-approved vaginal creams to help build up the vaginal skin (mucosa). They are Estrace Vaginal Cream and Premarin Vaginal Cream. The Estrace Vaginal Cream is estradiol cream. It contains one estrogen: estradiol. Premarin Vaginal Cream is what is called a conjugated estrogen cream. This means that there are several estrogens conjugated (or combined) together: estradiol, estriol, and estrone.

You get an applicator tube with the cream, but only about a half-inch (one to two grams) is needed in the tube. I like to show the tube in the exam room so that patients understand that it is just a small amount. The cream is formulated to adhere to the walls of the vagina and not leak out, but women find that any leakage is annoying. These creams are very expensive on some insurance plans.

The second option is a small vaginal pill that contains estradiol only. This pill is called Vagifem. It is only available in one dose in the United States. The pill comes in the top of a light blue applicator that is put into the vagina. The pill is released on the other end by "clicking" the pill into the vagina like clicking a ballpoint pen. This is by far the easiest and, in my opinion, the most frequent choice that patients choose. It is not messy (like the cream can be) and does not "leak out" of the vagina when you stand up.

The third option for vaginal (local) estrogen is the Estring vaginal ring. The Estring is approved for vaginal dryness. This is a very convenient way to get local estrogen if you do not mind sticking your fingers in your vagina to put it in or take it out. It is very easy to use. Once the package is opened, the estrogen is delivered right to the vagina from the ring; the medication lasts for three months. At the end of three months, you take it out and put in another. You can take it out every day if you want to wash it off and you can take it out for intercourse. It is a silastic ring impregnated with estradiol. You take it out of the package, squeeze it, and push it in as high as you can. The edge will rest on your pubic bone. For those of you who used a diaphragm many years ago, you put it in your vagina exactly the same way. I really have not had anyone have a bad reaction to vaginal estrogen. Some women may have vaginal irritation (possible allergic reaction to the cream), vaginal discharge, or breast tenderness. Usually women just cannot remember to use it regularly. However, I did get this call from a patient while she was on vacation: "I was put on estrogen vaginal cream at my last visit. We are on vacation and my husband's mouth is all broken out in a rash. What should we do?" Give him some Benadryl, put some hydrocortisone cream on it, and go to the hospital if his lips start to swell or he has trouble breathing. That would be a difficult thing to tell the ER doctor.

Vaginal estrogen is poorly absorbed into the body and does not stimulate other estrogen receptors—that is, in the breasts, uterus, and the brain. Some patients get breast tenderness on vaginal estrogen. It must be from the stimulation of estrogen receptors in their breasts. Can a patient with breast cancer go on vaginal estrogen? I think that the woman with breast cancer and severe vaginal dryness should talk to her oncologist and breast surgeon. Promptly those two physicians are then going to tell her that that is between her and her gynecologist. (No doctor wants to answer this question.) Do I know one hundred percent that it is not going to stimulate her breast cancer? Absolutely not. I would like her to wait until she is five years out from her last treatment. Why? It makes us feel better. This is uncomfortable for all of her physicians. If the patient was on an anti-estrogen such as Tamoxifen for five years, it is a little absurd to put her back on estrogen. Then I am the one that put her back on estrogen. I know that it is not supposed to cause any systemic effects; but remember that your doctor is also upset when something goes wrong. We hate to have a bad outcome as much as the patient and the family. How do you think I would feel if I had prescribed it and then she had a recurrence of her breast cancer? On the other hand, if she comes into the office and has finally finished all her chemotherapy and radiation and has been cancer free but has severe pain with intercourse and wants to get back to normal, do I deny her the one medication that may improve her sex life because I do not want the worry? There is a new oral medication for vaginal dryness called Osphena. The generic name is ospemifene. It was developed for vaginal dryness. Per the package insert, the first and only FDA-approved non-estrogen oral treatment reverses certain physical changes of the vagina and significantly relieves moderate to severe painful intercourse due to menopause.

How does it work? Well, the medication works by binding to the estrogen receptors.

As you know by now, estrogen receptors are in many places. They are in your brain, your breasts, your genital regions, and in your uterus. The company has made this drug stimulate only your vaginal estrogen receptors (what we call an "agonist" response) while blocking other estrogen receptors (an "antagonist" response). The idea is very good. If this drug stimulates only vaginal estrogen receptors, it would stimulate your vaginal tissues to become thick, well lubricated, and will keep those "folds" present. Again, the folds in your vagina (the rugae), keep the vagina mobile like an accordion. It stretches out and shrinks back up. These folds are imperative to maintain so that pain with intercourse does not occur. The idea for the drug is brilliant. The problem is that they cannot exclusively stimulate only the vaginal receptors perfectly. Per the Osphena pamphlet, taking Osphena may increase your chance of getting cancer of the lining of the uterus (the endometrial lining), but this risk is very low. In addition, Osphena may increase your chance of suffering from strokes and blood clots and has the same effect on promoting blood clots. Therefore, it is not perfect; but it is the best we have at this point for a non-hormonal treatment for vaginal dryness. It is a new drug, so we will see how people respond. At this point it is not indicated for use in women with breast cancer.

I hope that those clinical trials will be done, because vaginal dryness is the number one complaint of women being treated for breast cancer. I wish that the company had done the clinical trials to approve the drug in women with breast cancer. Just like men having multiple medical problems that affect the small blood vessels in their penises, women can have small blood vessels in the vagina be affected as well. As we age, other health problems can decrease blood supply to the area, such as hypertension, high cholesterol, heart disease, smoking, and diabetes. Make sure that you are getting your annual exams and checking your blood pressure, cholesterol, and sugar levels. Smoking causes damage to all small blood vessels. You cannot live in America and not know how dangerous smoking is to your health. If you are smoking, please stop. If you do not smoke, please do not start.

36
SYSTEMIC ESTROGEN

In the 1940's a Canadian drug maker found a way to isolate estrogen from pregnant horse (mare) urine. The drug, aptly called Premarin stands for *Pre*gnant *Ma*re Ur*ine*. Premarin was found to help women with hot flashes. At the time, drug makers had to prove only that the drug posed no immediate danger to the user. In the 1950's the makers of Premarin promoted it as a rejuvenating agent and mood stabilizer for postmenopausal women. By the mid-1960's about 12 percent of all postmenopausal women were taking the drug.

In the 1960's pharmaceutical companies had to prove the effectiveness of a drug before it reached market by performing clinical trials. These trials only had to go on for twelve to twenty-four months. It was not until the 1990's that researchers started getting interested in the long-term effects of estrogen therapy. Systemic estrogen that goes all through your body, such as pills, the Femring vaginal ring, patches, gels, creams, and pellets, are also an option to stimulate the estrogen receptors in your vagina. The problem is that they also stimulate the estrogen receptors all over your body, especially your breasts. For women who have vaginal dryness and hot flashes, you can use a systemic estrogen. If you only have symptoms of vaginal dryness, then there is no reason to take systemic estrogen. In fact, it would be foolish to take the risk if you were not having any problems with hot flashes. The risks associated with these estrogens are much greater.

The following safety information is given to physicians (and hopefully) patients when they are put on estrogen replacement therapy.

Warning: endometrial cancer, cardiovascular disorders, breast cancer, and probably dementia. See full prescribing information for complete boxed warning.

Estrogen-Alone Therapy

There is an increased risk of endometrial cancer in a woman with a uterus who uses unopposed estrogens. Estrogen-alone therapy should not be used for the prevention of cardiovascular disease or dementia. The Women's Health Initiative (WHI) estrogen-alone sub-study reported increased risks of stroke and deep vein thrombosis (DVT). The WHI Memory Study (WHIMS) estrogen-alone ancillary study of WHI reported an increased risk of probable dementia in postmenopausal women sixty-five years of age or older.

Estrogen, plus progestin, therapy

Estrogen, plus progestin, therapy should not be used for the prevention of cardio-vascular disease or dementia. The WHI estrogen, plus progestin, sub-study reported increased risks of DVT, pulmonary embolism (PE), stroke, and myocardial infarction (MI). The WHI estrogen, plus progestin, sub-study reported increased risks of invasive breast cancer. The WHIMS estrogen, plus progestin, ancillary study of WHI reported an increased risk of probable dementia in postmenopausal women sixty-five years of age or older.

After reading this, anybody would be too scared to take this medication. The above statements are very scary for patients and physicians. As a physician, I try to put these sentences in perspective when I am recommending or offering estrogen therapy. I think that all OB/GYN physicians would like to explain this "safety information" in detail to their patients. There just is not the time during a fifteen-minute or twenty-minute time slot to cover this appropriately and get to all the other things that you need to talk about, let alone leaving time for the exam. Do some physicians just not talk about it because they do not want to take the medical and legal risks? Probably. Do some of them not talk about it because they do not have the time? Yes.

It is probably easier to tell the patient that the risks are the risks and take them if you want; this would save time and potential medical and legal problems. I am going to give you my spiel that I would like to tell every patient in the office if I had an unlimited amount of time.

Prior to 2001, I was a foot-stomping, evangelical, hormone replacement therapy (HRT) giver. At the time, we thought that starting hormones (estrogen and progesterone) right at the beginning of menopause would help prevent the aging of the skin that occurs when your ovaries fail. It probably does. Women who menstruate longer look younger to me. Sometimes when someone is over fifty-one or so and does not look their age, I ask if they are still menstruating. They usually are surprised by the question and say, "Yes, how did you know?" I usually tell them because their skin looks good and has fewer wrinkles than I would expect. We thought that giving HRT at the time of menopause prevented heart disease in women. This was because of the observation that men had more heart disease than women did, but after menopause, women caught up with the men. These data were wrong. We thought that HRT that was started at the time of menopause helped to prevent memory loss. These data are wrong. It appears that it may increase the risk of dementia in women over the age of sixty-five. We also thought that starting HRT that at the time of menopause prevented bone loss. It does, but it is not worth the risk of a heart attack, stroke, or pulmonary embolus. The drug Fosamax, which is used to reverse bone loss, came out around 1999. So, before that the only thing that we could do to help stop bone loss was to prescribe estrogen. What did we know back then about HRT? We knew that there might be an association with breast cancer, and we knew that it could cause blood clots. We knew that these blood clots could break off and travel to other parts of the body, including the lungs. This is called a pulmonary embolus and can be fatal. Why did we prescribe it prior to 2001? Well, one in three women were dying of heart disease and one in eight women developed breast cancer. We had nothing but estrogen to prevent osteoporosis and, at the time, 50 to 80 percent of women died within two years of breaking their hips. We thought it helped with the effects of aging and memory loss. We knew that if a woman had a uterus, they had to take the sister-hormone progesterone to prevent uterine cancer. We knew that estrogens might increase gallbladder disease. We knew that estrogen helped with vaginal atrophy and prevented pain with intercourse after menopause. We thought that the benefits outweighed the risks.

I once heard a medical student ask one of my OB/GYN professors how long a woman should take HRT. He said, "You should slip the last one between her teeth as they are lowering her into the ground." This may sound cavalier, but if you think about how many men and women are on drugs for cholesterol, it would make your head spin. Cholesterol drugs give a great example of risk: benefit ratios of drugs. At this time in medicine it has been shown repeatedly in clinical studies that if we keep a patient's cholesterol down, their risk of dying from a heart attack and stroke plummets. However, these cholesterol drugs, commonly called "statins," can cause fatal liver failure. If you get liver failure, you are not going to make it. You must go into the office at least every six months and get blood work to check your liver. If we find liver problems early, we can stop the medication, and your liver should heal. If you do not come in and get the labs and your liver is failing, you can die. So do not give your doctor a hard time about coming in for labs. We do not want to be responsible for your death because you did not have the time to come in for lab work.

So what happened with hormone replacement therapy? Well, in 2001 a study came out on the news. This study was called the Women's Health Initiative. The problem with the study was not in its design, but the way that the results were reported. For the first time in my years as a physician, the world got the results before the medical profession. Usually the results come out in a reputable medical journal and physicians around the world have a chance to review the work, analyze the data, and discuss the results. In this case the study was first reported on the nightly news weeks before the journal was even supposed to be in the mail. In their usual "breaking news alert" fashion, the world was told that estrogen replacement therapy causes breast cancer. The physicians in this country and around the world had patients calling our offices asking about the results of this study. No one could respond because no one had the journal. The usual reporting protocol had been bypassed and physicians, especially OB/GYNs, looked incredibly stupid. We could not answer the questions that the news anchors asked. Subsequently, many women in the United States abruptly stopped their hormone replacement therapy, having been frightened out of their minds that they would get breast cancer. It took a while for the medical community to do what they usually do prior to this type of report. It took several months for physicians to read the article, critique the data, and discuss the results. Now, at this point, you may think that I really hate this study. I don't.

This study came out in the *Journal of the American Medical Association* (JAMA), which is one of the most reputable medical journals in the world. The study that was performed was a randomized, double-blind, placebo-controlled experiment. This means that the physicians and researchers as well as the patients did not know who was on a placebo or the real drug. It is the best study that you can do to answer a clinical question about a drug. I cannot emphasize enough that the study design was perfect. They put thousands of women on hormone replacement therapy and thousands of women on placebo drugs. The study was stopped when the computer analysis showed that more patients got breast cancer when they were on the hormones. There is no doubt that the results were real. However, if you look at it from a gynecologist's perspective, do you really think the patients did not know that they were on hormones?

The only way to carry out this study correctly was to pick women that had no menopausal symptoms. If they had any symptoms at all, they had to have known that they were not taking a placebo, because their symptoms would have gone away. That is just what these researchers did; they chose patients who had no menopausal symptoms at all. On average, the patients were sixty-three years of age at the start of the study. The problem with the clinical usefulness of this study is that no gynecologist is going to put their patient on hormone replacement therapy at sixty-three years of age with no menopausal symptoms. It would be like putting a patient on cholesterol medication that did not have high cholesterol. Why would you risk giving someone liver failure when they did not need the medication? You wouldn't. The patients that we were putting on hormone replacement therapy were symptomatic and usually were at the beginning of menopause.

Let us pretend that you, the reader of this passage, are the doctor and I am your patient. If I came into your office and said, "Doctor, my friend Sally is on hormone replacement therapy, and she is really happy. I want you to give me some of the hormones that she is taking so that I can be as happy as she is," you, as the physician, should say, "Are you having any hot flashes, night sweats, or vaginal dryness?" If I replied, "No, I just want to be as happy she is," then you should refuse to give me the medication. A physician would not put an asymptomatic patient on a drug that could potentially hurt them. Hormone replacement therapy should be given to women whose quality of life *without hormones* is worse than the risk she has accepted by taking them. We put patients on the lowest possible dose of hormone for the shortest period that they need them. Periodically we try to have the patient wean off the hormones to see how they do on lower doses. Eventually most patients can wean off these drugs. What they did not report on the nightly news is that there are subsets of this study. As I indicated, there were those patients that were taking placebos and those that were taking hormones. If you have a uterus, you have to take the sister-hormone progesterone with the estrogen to prevent a buildup of tissue inside the uterus. The buildup of this tissue can turn into uterine cancer. If patients do not have a uterus, then they do not need the progesterone. The nightly news anchors did not tell the world that the only patients who developed breast cancer in higher amounts than the placebos were the ones that were taking estrogen and progesterone. The patients who did not have a uterus and were only taking estrogen did not have an increase in breast cancer. In fact, that study is still going on and they still have not had an increase in breast cancer in these women taking estrogen only. What does this mean for the patient? It must make you ask the question, "Is it the progesterone that is causing the cancer?" I don't know. Maybe.

Therefore, when I have a patient that needs estrogen replacement therapy but does not have a uterus, I do not give her progesterone. Many women read on the

Internet that progesterone cream can help women feel better during menopause. When they ask me about this, I explain the results of this study. If it were me, I would not take progesterone orally or topically because of the results of this study. If you do not have a uterus, why would you take it? I wouldn't.

37
REEVALUATION OF THE WARNINGS

Now that you know about the Women's Health Initiative Study, I would like to take the "Important Safety Information" statements that are in every estrogen package one by one. They will make much more sense to you now. I have put the statements in italics and my responses to the statements below the statement.

Warning: Endometrial cancer, cardiovascular disorders, breast cancer, and probable dementia.

The above statement warns that estrogen can cause endometrial cancer. We know that if you take estrogen without progesterone when you have a uterus, it increases the risk of endometrial cancer; therefore, we do not give estrogen-replacement therapy without the sister-hormone progesterone in patients that have a uterus. There is a risk of heart attack when taking estrogen-replacement therapy because one of the risks of estrogen is blood clots. These blood clots can break off and travel to your head causing a stroke, to your lungs causing a pulmonary embolus, or to your heart causing a heart attack. The Women's Health Initiative Study did show an increase in breast cancers (eight more patients per ten thousand total patients) in the group that took estrogen and progesterone. The Women's Health Initiative Study also showed that there was a possible increase in dementia in women who took estrogen.

Estrogen-Alone Therapy

This section applies to only the women in the study that took estrogen alone. This arm of the study only included women who did not have a uterus.

There is an increased risk of endometrial cancer in a woman with a uterus who uses unopposed estrogens.

OB/GYNs are well aware that if you give women with a uterus estrogen without progesterone they can get endometrial cancer.

Estrogen-alone therapy should not be used for the prevention of cardiovascular disease or dementia.

The Women's Health Initiative did show us that estrogen could cause heart attacks and dementia. However, this was not an indication that we used to put people on estrogen. The main diagnosis to put a woman on systemic estrogen is menopausal symptoms, that is, hot flashes, mood swings, night sweats, and vaginal dryness.

The Women's Health Initiative (WHI) estrogen-alone sub-study reported increased risks of stroke and deep vein thrombosis (DVT).

Long before the Women's Health Initiative Study, physicians knew, and especially OB/GYNs knew, that estrogen increased the risk of blood clots (deep vein thrombosis or DVT) which leads to an increased risk of stroke.

The WHI Memory Study (WHIMS) estrogen-alone ancillary study of WHI reported an increased risk of probable dementia in postmenopausal women sixty-five years of age or older.

Physicians, and especially OB/GYNs, did not know that there is an increased risk of probable dementia in women who are over sixty-five years of age and who take estrogen. However, you do not have to be a physician to know that all people can get dementia, and the older you are the more likely you are to have dementia. Remember, we do not usually give estrogen-replacement therapy to women who have no menopausal symptoms (especially over sixty-five); we would never give estrogen to someone to prevent dementia.

Estrogen Plus Progestin Therapy

This section applies to only the women in the study that took estrogen and progesterone. This arm of the study only included women who did have a uterus.

Estrogen plus progestin therapy should not be used for the prevention of cardiovascular disease or dementia.

The Women's Health Initiative did show us that estrogen plus progesterone could cause heart attacks and dementia. However, this was not an indication that we used to put people on estrogen. The main diagnosis to put a woman on systemic estrogen is menopausal symptoms—that is, hot flashes, mood swings, night sweats, and vaginal dryness.

The WHI estrogen plus progestin sub-study reported increased risks of DVT, pulmonary embolism (PE), stroke, and myocardial infarction (MI).

Long before the Women's Health Initiative Study, physicians knew, and especially OB/GYNs knew, that estrogen increased the risk of blood clots (deep vein thrombosis or DVT), which leads to an increased risk of stroke. Could the progesterone be causing the increase in pulmonary embolus (PE) and heart attack (MI)?

Did you notice that the pulmonary embolus and the myocardial infarction (heart attack, MI) risks were not reported in the patients taking estrogen only?

The WHI estrogen plus progestin sub-study reported increased risks of invasive breast cancer.

The Women's Health Initiative Study did show an increase in invasive breast cancer in women taking estrogen plus progesterone. Did you notice that in women taking estrogen only there was no increase in invasive breast cancer? Could it be the progesterone?

The WHIMS estrogen plus progestin ancillary study of WHI reported an increased risk of probable dementia in postmenopausal women sixty-five years of age or older.

Physicians, and especially OB/GYNs, did not know that there is an increased risk of probable dementia in women who are over sixty-five years of age and who take estrogen. However, you do not have to be a physician to know that all people can get dementia, and the older you are the more likely you are to have dementia. Remember, we do not usually give estrogen replacement therapy to women that have no menopausal symptoms (especially over sixty-five); we would never give estrogen to someone to prevent dementia.

So, as you can see, without having the journal article for at least a month after this was reported on the nightly news, physicians could not evaluate and respond to our patient's questions. I am not disputing the results of the study at all; this was an extremely well-done study, and in order to get accurate results, they had to include women that were older and were not menopausal. However, these patients are not the ones who are prescribed estrogen.

At any rate, millions of women stopped taking their hormone replacement therapy because of the increased risk of breast cancer. Because the results of the study were not known to the general physician population, millions of women who were not taking progesterone because they did not have a uterus also stopped their hormones. As you can see, this discussion is very difficult to have at the time of the annual examination when you only have a brief period in which to get everything done. There is no way to explain this study to every menopausal woman who walks in the door. I am sure that most OB/GYNs try to summarize this; however, it probably comes across as confusing and ultimately dangerous to take the drug. Overall, the results of the Women's Health Initiative Study can be summarized as follows.

For every ten thousand women who take Prempro (the estrogen/progesterone drug used for the study), compared with women who do not, annually there will be: eight more cases of breast cancer, six more heart attacks, seven more strokes, eighteen more life-threatening blood clots, five fewer hip fractures, and six fewer cases of colon cancer.

38
HOW DOES YOUR OB/GYN REALLY FEEL ABOUT ESTROGEN?

I like to tell the following story. In 2006 I was attending the Georgia OB/GYN Society meeting at a fancy beach resort. That year I was the president-elect of the society. That means that the following year, I was going to be president. My late husband and I were attending the second-to-the-last talk of the morning. The lectures usually stopped about one o'clock, and then we would be free to enjoy the resort at our leisure until the evening activities began. The last talk of the morning was on hormone replacement therapy. (Oh my God, not again.)

My children were upstairs in our hotel room waiting for us to finish our lecture series so that we could take them to the beach. During the break between lectures, I leaned over and told my husband that we needed to leave. I said, "Let's get out of here. I cannot stand to hear one more lecture on hormone therapy and how bad it is for my patients. Let's go get the kids and go to the beach." He said to me, "Pam, you can't leave; it will look terrible if you leave. How can you walk out on the last lecture when you are going to be the president of the society next year? It will look terrible."

Well, he made me feel bad enough that I stayed, but I was not happy about it. My fears were confirmed exponentially when this man walked up to the podium with big black-rimmed eyeglasses. He shuffled his notes around like the absent-minded professor who did not have his papers in order. He stuttered, apologized, and proceeded to start the most boring lecture on hormones that I have ever heard. He talked in a monotone voice and never looked at the audience or pointed to his slides. For about eight minutes he went over all the bad things that hormone replacement therapy can cause.

Just shoot me. I rolled my eyes at my husband; he knew that he was going to pay for this. I was thinking that I deserved a new bathing suit for the beach. At about ten minutes into his lecture, the lecturer stopped talking, threw his big eyeglasses down on the podium, took off his coat and tie, and exclaimed, "Please let me talk about what is great about hormone placement therapy." Everyone in the room was in shock. You have to understand that at medical seminars the audience is quite reserved. We come dressed in business attire and maintain a professional air about the lecture room. It is very unusual for anyone to jump up and down and yell, especially the lecturer. Then, in a very excited and "pumped-up" fashion, he talked about the benefits of hormone replacement therapy. He talked about how great women looked when they took estrogen at the beginning of menopause. He talked about how happy they were. He talked about their lack of mood swings. He lectured extensively about the positive effects on bone to prevent osteoporosis and the positive effects on the vagina, which prevented the vaginal dryness, atrophy, and pain with intercourse. He was literally jumping up and down and banging his fist on the podium while he was talking about the effect on hot flashes, night sweats, and insomnia. There were 130 OB/GYN physicians in that audience and everybody was smiling. At this point, I thought, this has to be one of the best lectures I have ever heard on any topic in my life. (I also realized that I didn't deserve, and definitely wasn't going to get, my new bathing suit.)

I will never forget the last sentence of his lecture. He jumped up in the air with his arms above his head, came down, and hit both fists on the podium. He looked out at the audience and said, "Let's feel good about making our patients feel good. Let's give them their estrogen back." Well, if you had been there you could have seen 130 physicians jump out of their seats screaming, hollering, clapping, and whistling. It was the only time in my medical career that I have seen this at a meeting. He got a standing ovation for about ten minutes. I wish I had a video of the last two minutes of his lecture; I wish that patients could really see how their OB/GYN may feel about this problem. I wish that our patients knew how much we wanted to help them, but at the same time, not hurt them. It is a difficult balance to maintain.

Do I personally believe that hormone replacement therapy is good? There is no way to answer this. I know that it makes many women feel good. Each patient has to be looked at separately. Each woman has to evaluate just how bad she feels during her menopausal years, what her family history has been, and how scared she is to take the drug. If she has a mother and grandmother with breast cancer, then it may not be a great idea. If everyone in your family has died of strokes or heart attacks, you have to evaluate the risks with your physician. What if she brings three changes of clothes to work and cannot function because of hot flashes? So many things in medicine do not have a "right" answer; the patient must be fully informed and actively participate in the decisions regarding their health care. In cases like this—that is, taking a drug that may be dangerous—the patient must take responsibility for their own health care. The physician must take responsibility for providing all the information that the patient needs to make a decision accurately and in a way that the patient understands. As I indicated before, there is just not enough time in a normal visit to go through all of the risks, caveats, worries, and benefits.

39
WHICH HORMONE SHOULD YOU TAKE?

Once you have made the decision to take systemic hormones, which ones do you take? There are many different brands. Are any of them safer? There is no right answer. A physician must individually assess each patient. The following is the spiel that I give my patients. Now that you have made the decision ("informed consent" is the proper medical term), to start systemic estrogen, I would like you to try the transdermal (topical or placed on the skin) estrogens as opposed to oral estrogen. There are several reasons why I start with the topical estrogens. When you put the estrogen on your skin, the drug does not go through (get filtered by) your liver. For several reasons, this is a safer administration of the drug than taking a pill. Oral estrogens can increase triglyceride (fat) levels in your blood, which we do not want to do after menopause. Remember, one in three women will die of heart disease, so it is very important to keep your cholesterol and triglyceride levels within normal range. It has been clinically proven in multiple studies that if your cholesterol and triglyceride levels stay within the normal ranges, you have a significantly decreased risk of having a heart attack or a stroke. Oral estrogens also increase a substance in your blood stream called sex-hormone binding globulin (SHBG).

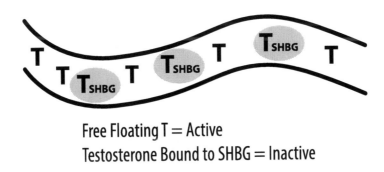

Free Floating T = Active
Testosterone Bound to SHBG = Inactive

SHBG binds to free-floating testosterone in the bloodstream and makes it inactive, it does not work anymore. Only unbound, free-floating testosterone is active.

Theoretically this will lower your libido. With the lack of libido problem that occurs in menopause, we really do not want to add to the problem of low testosterone by giving you a drug that lowers your free-floating testosterone. The free-floating testosterone is the one that makes you want to have sex. It makes you horny.

There is also the same effect on your thyroid binding globulin (TBG). Every menopausal woman who walks into my office and who has weight gain desperately wants to have low thyroid levels to explain it. Most of them do not have low thyroid levels. When we check thyroid levels, we want you to have a normal level of thyroxine (also called T4). Oral estrogen increases the level of thyroid binding globulin, which binds to the thyroxine (T4) that is floating freely and makes it inactive. Theoretically this could slow down your metabolism and add to weight gain. Again, it just seems counterintuitive to give it orally when we are giving the estrogen to help you with menopausal symptoms. The last reason to give the estrogen topically is that the risk of blood clots and stroke appears to be higher with oral estrogens. Is this because it can increase your triglyceride levels? Probably. We just do not want to take the chance if we do not have to. There are many types of transdermal estrogen:

Gels: Elestrin, Divigel, and Estrogel.

Cream: Estrasorb.

Topical spray: Evamist.

Vaginal estrogen: Femring (this gives a higher dose than the Estring that is used for vaginal dryness and atrophy).

Topical patches that have estrogen only: Minivelle, Climara, Estraderm, Alora, Menostar.

Topical patches that have estrogen and progesterone: Combipatch, Climarapro.

The consensus among OB/GYNs is to start on the lowest dose and work up until a patient's symptoms have stopped. It is recommended to increase the dose monthly. It is felt that this approach is associated with less vaginal bleeding and breast tenderness. I personally find that this approach just pisses my patients off. I give every one of them the option of starting low and then working their way up or starting high and weaning them to a lower dose. Almost all of my patients choose to start high and wean down. This is almost certainly because of how I present the data to them, and I understand that. The problem is that my patients are happier when I take care of their symptoms quickly. I think that they do better this way, and my patients have been counseled on the fact that they may have more breast tenderness and/or vaginal bleeding if they do it this way. These symptoms usually get better in a few weeks to months. It is a small price to pay if they are finally sleeping through the night. It may be worth it to a specific patient if she is not changing clothes three times a day because of hot flashes. It may benefit society if a woman is not thinking of ways to kill people who piss them off. The next question that they are going to ask me is, "When are we going to check my hormone levels?" Ugh. I know that sometimes I get frustrated with this question, and before I answer, I acknowledge this to my patient. It is very common for women to go to physicians who check many blood levels of the common hormones. This can get very expensive, as many insurance companies do not pay for this testing. I hear about these patients going back every three months to check the levels. I do not refuse to check levels if the patient would like them checked. I do, however, let them know that it is usually expensive, and I am not sure of what benefit it is to check them. The North American Menopause Society does not recommend testing levels of hormones. I agree completely.

If you are coming to me with severe menopausal symptoms and have not had a period in fifteen months, I can tell you what your estrogen and progesterone levels are going to be: they are low. If you are still having a period, but are having hot flashes and night sweats, the levels are going to be normal. I am going to offer to put both of these patients on hormone replacement therapy no matter what their levels are. I am treating your symptoms, not your lab results. If they are put on the HRT and come back in a month and are very happy, I am going to start weaning them down. I have them take a lower dose every one to two months until their symptoms return. I have them stay on the dose where they were the happiest. I then see them every six months to a year, and we talk about decreasing the dose. I have my patients try to wean off their hormones at least once a year. If the patient is happy and her hormone level is low, should I increase it just to get a good lab level? Of course not.

We want you on the lowest possible dose for the shortest period of time. Now, every physician has their way of doing things. There are going to be some OB/GYNs who completely disagree with my approach. My approach is not wrong, and their approach is not wrong. The practice of medicine is just that. Practice. Unfortunately we practice on our patients until we get it right, for us *and* for our patients. The most important thing is keeping the patient informed. They must be kept part of the decision-making process, but we cannot let the patient make decisions that can hurt them. Some physicians give injectable estrogen (into the muscle) and implantable estrogen (pellets placed into the fat of their abdomen) for hormone replacement. I do not stop my patients from having these types of administration of estrogen, but I do not do it. It is reasonable to check estrogen levels in these patients, because the level may get significantly high. The patients tend to get a steroid "high" after the administration and then, as it wears off, they report a "crash" if they do not get the dose given again in the appropriate amount of time. Several physicians in my city are comfortable giving estrogen in this fashion. I am not comfortable with it, and therefore I do not do it. It does not make me angry or uncomfortable if they go to another physician to get it administered in that fashion. I do make sure that they are on the sister-hormone progesterone if they have a uterus.

There are several oral estrogens:

Oral estradiol: Estrace.

Oral esterified estrogen: Menest.

Oral estropipate: Ortho-Est.

Oral Conjugated estrogens: Premarin.

Oral conjugated synthetic estrogens: Cenestin, Enjuvia.

Oral estrogen-progesterone combinations: Prempro, Prefest, Activella, Mimvey, Jinteli, Angeliq.

HERBS, OPTIONS, PILLS, LUBES, AND TUBES

40
Herbal Alternatives

A number of herbal treatments have been promoted as a "natural" remedy for hot flashes. It is estimated that 50 to 75 percent of postmenopausal women use alternative therapies for menopausal symptoms, especially women with breast cancer. In fact, many postmenopausal women use black cohosh for hot flashes, but clinical trials have shown that it is only as effective as a placebo. In addition, there are some safety issues about some herbs, including black cohosh, which might stimulate breast tissue (similar to estrogen). Herbal treatments are not recommended for hot flashes or other menopausal symptoms. However, if you are taking herbal treatments and your symptoms are relieved by this treatment, then *no one* will be happier than I will. I would rather not have you on systemic estrogen; it can be dangerous. Are you getting better because of the 30 percent placebo effect that occurs with all drugs? Are you getting better because it is really helping your symptoms? A new medication is sold over the counter for hot flashes that is a Swedish flower pollen extract. The pollen allergens have been removed, and it is grown without pesticides. There are clinical studies that show the effectiveness of this medication. You can read about this at www.relizen.com or on Facebook at Facebook.com/RelizenMenopause. You can also call Relizen toll-free at 1-855-RE-LIZEN to order the pills over the phone. Other alternatives which have helped some women are paced respiration, mind-body therapies (deep breathing exercises and guided imagery), weight loss, exercise, acupuncture, evening primrose oil, flaxseed, mindfulness training, hypnosis, and cognitive behavioral therapy.

41
Phytoestrogens and Bio-Identical Hormones

Phytoestrogens are non-steroidal compounds that occur naturally in many plants, fruits, and vegetables. There are three main types of phytoestrogens: isoflavones (genistein, and daidzein), coumestans, and lignans (enterolactone and enterodiol). Two types of isoflavones, genistein and daidzein, are found in soybeans, chickpeas, and lentils, and are thought to be the most potent estrogens of the phytoestrogens (although, they are less potent than estradiol).

Lignans (enterolactone and enterodiol) are found in flaxseed, lentils, grains, fruits, and vegetables. It has been suggested that the lower risk of heart disease among Asian people compared with western people is due to the high consumption of soybean products. Because of this observation, many have looked into using phytoestrogens as an alternative to hormone therapy for postmenopausal women. In fact, a high percentage of women (including women with a history of breast cancer) use soy in their diets to help with hot flashes. Many women perceive that phytoestrogens, because they are "natural," are safer than standard FDA-approved estrogens. This has never been proven.

The studies on phytoestrogens to treat hot flashes are not conclusive at all. Most studies have not shown them to help with these symptoms. A review of seventy-four studies of phytoestrogens in humans concluded that "while evidence for the potential health benefits of phytoestrogens is increasing, it is still insufficient to recommend them in place of traditional hormone replacement therapy."

The "bio-identical" approach generally refers to doctors prescribing estrogens, progesterones, and testosterone in individual doses. They are put together or "compounded" as pills, gels, under-the-tongue tablets, or suppositories. Many women assume that "natural" hormones are safer. They are not. Bio-identical hormones are identical in molecular structure to the hormones women make in their bodies. They are made from a plant chemical taken out of yams and soy. The bioidentical estrogens are: 17-beta-estradiol, estrone, and estriol.

The quality of compounded products may be below standards at many pharmacies. In one study, potencies ranged from 67 percent to 268 percent of the amount specified on the labeling. The hormones most commonly compounded are: estradiol, estrone, estriol, progesterone, testosterone, and dehydroepiandrosterone (DHEA).

Women typically are asked to submit saliva, urine, or blood samples to measure hormone levels. Once the results are reported, the physician picks the doses of hormones to give that particular patient. Unfortunately, these results do not help much because there is no data to support that hormone levels in saliva, urine, or blood correlates to treatment success. Those who push bio-identical hormones claim that these hormones are better for menopausal symptoms and are safer and better tolerated than FDA-approved hormones. However, a review of the literature concluded: "While some of these products may decrease hot flushes, there is no evidence that "bio-identical" hormones have any advantage over conventional hormone therapies." The U.S. Food and Drug Administration (FDA) has published consumer information warning consumers: "Many claims made about the safety and efficacy of compounded bio-identical hormone products are false and misleading, with no credible scientific evidence to support them." In a 2006 position statement that was reissued in 2009, the Endocrine Society stated: "There is no scientific evidence to support the efficacy, safety, or effectiveness of compounded bio-identical hormones."

Now, after I discuss this with my patients, and they decide that they want the bio-identical prescription, I will give it to them. I document this discussion in the chart. Insurance companies do not cover the cost of bio-identical hormones. In addition to their insurance premiums, many women pay a hundred dollars a month or more for these hormones. If it were me, I would try the FDA approved ones first so that my insurance would pay for it.

42

PROGESTERONES

Endometrial hyperplasia (overgrowth of the lining of the uterus) and cancer can occur after as little as six months if a woman with a uterus uses estrogen without progesterone. So progesterones should be added in women who have not had a hysterectomy. Women who have undergone a hysterectomy should not receive progesterone. The most commonly prescribed progesterone to use with estrogen replacement is Provera, or medroxyprogesterone acetate (MPA). Most physicians are going to prescribe this daily at a low dose (2.5 mg) that has been proven in clinical studies to prevent endometrial cancer. Some women (who like to have a period each month) take it in a cyclic fashion; they take 10 mg for ten to twelve days each month. Because the progesterone is withdrawn each month, the patient experiences the withdrawal of progesterone, which makes the blood come out. This is not a "period." This bleeding has nothing to do with your ovaries. We are just withdrawing the progesterone, and the uterus will now have a withdrawal of the blood lining.

Prometrium is progesterone that is a natural oral-micronized progesterone. It has been proven to protect the endometrial lining from cancer and is associated with less vaginal bleeding. The usual dose is 200 mg/day cyclically for twelve days (if you want to bleed) or 200 mg/day continuously (so that you do not have a withdrawal bleed). Although it has been less well studied than Provera, it is a reasonable choice for women who cannot tolerate Provera. One may start with Provera as the progestin, particularly if cost is an issue; it is inexpensive. Prometrium may have advantages in some women, as it is less likely to increase cholesterol and triglycerides. The other thing to know is that, although data are limited, Prometrium may have less of an effect on breast cancer risk. Remember, based on the reports in the Women's Health Initiative Study, it may be the progesterone causing the breast cancer.

The Mirena IUD has been discussed in a previous chapter. Progesterone-releasing IUD is prescribed for birth control. Many physicians prescribe a Mirena IUD as an alternative for oral progesterone. The Mirena IUD is not FDA-approved for this use. The strategy is to avoid the possible increased risk of heart disease and breast cancer associated with systemic progesterones such as Provera and

Prometrium. I personally feel that the bleeding abnormalities are less with the Mirena IUD, it is one less pill to take, the patients do not feel that "PMS" feeling that progesterone gives they when you are taking them orally, and it lasts for five years! The Mirena IUD gives plenty of intrauterine progesterone (where you need it), but low systemic concentrations of progesterone (where you do not need it). Almost all women develop a very thin uterine lining or they do not have a lining at all (nothing to bleed). Awesome.

Something New
There is a new drug available from Pfizer Pharmaceuticals that is an alternative to taking progesterone with estrogen. The trade name is Duavee and is a prescription medication indicated for the treatment of hot flashes in women with a uterus. It contains a mixture of estrogens (conjugated estrogens) and bazedoxifene. Bazedoxifene is an estrogen agonist/antagonist that stops the estrogen lining on the uterus. I know that this is confusing, but the bazedoxifene is used *instead* of the progesterone. Duovee has estrogen; therefore, it still has all the side effects of estrogen. This would be a good alternative for a woman that had side effects from progesterone.

43
MALE HORMONES

Do women make male hormones? Yes. They are called androgens. The major androgens in women are dehydroepiandrosterone sulfate (DHEAS), dehydroepiandrosterone (DHEA), androstenedione (A), testosterone (T), and dihydrotestosterone (DHT).

They are listed in descending order of serum concentrations in premenopausal women.

Substance	Source	Percentage
DHEA-S:	Adrenal gland	(100%)
DHEA:	Adrenal gland	(50%)
	Ovary	(20%)
	Other	(30%)
A:	Adrenal gland	(50%)
	Ovary	(50%)
T:	Adrenal gland	(25%)
	Ovary	(25%)
	Conversion of A	(50%)

As we age, the production of all of these androgens goes down. After menopause the main role of the ovary is androgen (male hormone) production. Remember, a menopausal woman has no more eggs; therefore, they are not making any more estrogen. What role do androgens play in females? We really don't know. The assertion that low androgen levels play a role in female sexual function is based upon the known role of androgens in male sexuality. It makes men horny, so it should make women horny. In studies that measure male hormone levels and sexual function (horniness) in women, the correlation between male hormone levels and sexual function is just not there. In addition, women with high male hormone syndromes—that is, polycystic ovarian syndrome or male hormone secreting tumors—do not experience sexual benefits. (They are not more horny). Women with low male hormone syndromes—that is, removal of both ovaries surgically, or diseases in which the adrenal gland does not work well—or with hypopituitarism (the pituitary gland does not work well), do not necessarily have poor sexual function or libido. The levels of male hormones in women are much lower than in men, and there are no clear lab values for this because we really do not know what levels are good in a female. Should we give women testosterone? It is a good question and very hard to answer. Blood androgen (male hormone) levels do not really correlate with sexual function in women. Testosterone therapy, however, has been shown to improve sexual function in some postmenopausal women when given in high enough doses to get blood concentrations to levels that are *higher than normal* for women. The long-term consequences of these high testosterone levels are unknown. There are no FDA-approved testosterone products for women in the United States. This means that the FDA does not think that it is safe to use testosterone in women.

In order to give testosterone to our patients, we must prescribe it "off-label" and through a compounding pharmacy. That means that women are using a drug without FDA approval and without all the safety measures and quality controls that manufacturers of pharmaceuticals have to abide by, and the insurance companies will not pay for it because it is off-label. For all these years, these women have been paying insurance premiums and paying cash outside of their prescription coverage for drugs that were approved for men. Does this make you angry? It should. The FDA feels that it is OK for men to take the risk, but will not allow women to make that decision. I have recently seen some commercials on television from attorneys advertising to contact them if a patient was placed on testosterone and suffered a heart attack, stroke, or died. Well, there are risks to taking any drug. When you take a medication, you should be informed of the complications that can occur when taking the medication. No one in my practice gets testosterone in any form without me personally going through each of these risks with her. The role of testosterone administration in healthy premenopausal women (before the onset of menopause) has not been well studied.

Androstenedione (an androgen precursor that is widely used and promoted as "Andro" in bodybuilding magazines) increases blood levels of testosterone in some men. When given to women, androstenedione increases blood levels of testosterone and estrone concentrations. What happens to sexual function or its male hormone side-effects in women are not known. DHEA supplementation appears to help with the increase in a sense of well-being. It helps your insulin work well to metabolize sugars, and prevents bone loss at the hip or femoral neck in women with low male hormone levels that are from the adrenal glands. DHEA supplementation has been promoted as beneficial therapy for older men and women. While there is a well-known decline in blood levels of DHEA and DHEA-S as we get older, the effects of supplementation in perimenopausal and postmenopausal women are not understood. DHEA supplementation in otherwise healthy perimenopausal or postmenopausal women does not appear to be beneficial. Most male hormones are changed into estrogens within your body. It is imperative for physicians to put women on progesterone therapy to counteract the conversion of testosterone to estrogen if the patient has a uterus (even if they are not on estrogen). Each patient must be individualized.

44
A Libido Pill for Women?

We have been taught since our sexual education in high school that "sex" is dirty and that we can catch a terrible or even deadly disease. We have been taught in our religious teachings about the immorality of sex, adultery, and sexual acts. When we first get married, there is what I like to call the "jungle sex" period of our lives. Why don't we have fun jungle sex during our entire relationships? Well, we are tired. Exhausted. We are focusing on our careers, starting a family, and paying bills. For some reason we feel that our relationship should take a back seat to all of this.

I read a book when I was pregnant called *Baby Wise*. In that book there was a chapter about having protected time each day to spend on the marriage relationship. This time was sacred, and the authors recommended that the children should be brought up to respect this daily marriage time. Just as if they understand that they have to be in a car seat in the car, they understand that thirty minutes or an hour, or whatever time you choose, is "mommy and daddy time." They are not to disturb you two while you take the time to reconnect after a busy day. I did not follow this advice personally, but now that my children are older, I wish that I had. When you have children, and especially when you work, you feel the need to spend every second of your remaining day giving quality time to them. We have been conditioned to have their day completely planned from morning until night, lest they get an opportunity to use alcohol or drugs or hang around with the wrong crowd. We do not put nearly as much effort into our romantic and intimate relationship as we do planning our children's day. Women come in every day and ask me for a libido pill. There finally is a drug approved by the FDA for low libido in women. Flibanserin is a new drug just recently approved for the treatment of hypoactive sexual desire disorder (HSDD) in woman. HSDD means a woman who is otherwise healthy has a lacking libido or a lack of sexual desire. Studies show that about 10 to 20 percent of women face this problem, and some say HSDD outnumbers men with sexual problems. Flibanserin is not a hormone. It increases dopamine and nor-adrenalin within the brain and decreases serotonin. This has a positive effect on a woman's sexual craving who was otherwise lacking in this area.

Flibanserin was resubmitted for approval to the FDA in early 2015. It was approved in August and was available for the public at the end of October 2015. I love to tell the story of how Flibanserin was "found." I must give some background first. Rogaine, or Minoxidil, is a drug for hair loss. Minoxidil was going through clinical trials as a new blood pressure medication. It did not work at all. It did not lower blood pressure in people who were hypertensive. However, many people grew hair. Therefore, the makers of the drug resubmitted it to the FDA for hair growth. They went through clinical trials as a new drug to grow hair. It works great for many people, men and women. It is so terrible as a blood pressure medication that Rogaine is now over-the-counter.

Fast forward to the last several years. Flibanserin was originally going through clinical trials on people as a drug for depression. It did not work that well for depression, so the study was stopped. When the researchers let these people know that the study was stopped, many women were very upset and so were their intimate partners. It was then that they realized that a "side effect" of Flibanserin was increased sexual desire in women. The drug was then resubmitted to the FDA for approval for a libido pill for women. The drug goes by a trade name of Addyi. The generic name for the drug is Flibanserin. It is not going to be a complete cure for low libido in women. There will not be as good a response to this drug like men have to Viagra, Cialis, or Levitra, and, unfortunately, the drug has some side effects that might be frightening for some women. Physicians and healthcare providers who prescribe the drug must be "certified" because of the risk that patients might develop low blood pressure and faint. The certification process involves reading some literature, answering some questions, and sending this documentation to the company. Interestingly, the pharmacies that dispense and sell Flibanserin must be certified as well. These pharmacies will only fill the prescription that is written by a certified prescriber. This will be electronically verified when the prescription is processed through the pharmacy's computer system. The goal of the certification of both prescribers and pharmacies is to prevent the increased risks of low blood pressure and fainting associated with Addyi due to an interaction with alcohol by ensuring that *prescribers and pharmacists* are educated about the increased risk of low blood pressure and fainting associated with Addyi due to an interaction with alcohol and the need to counsel patients about this risk. It also informs *patients* of the increased risk of low blood pressure and fainting associated with Addyi due to an interaction with alcohol.

Addyi is indicated for the treatment of premenopausal women with acquired generalized Hypoactive Sexual Desire Disorder (HSDD) as characterized by low sexual desire that causes marked distress or interpersonal difficulty. The hypoactive sexual desire disorder *cannot* be due to a coexisting medical or psychiatric condition, problems within the relationship, the effects of a medication or other drug substance.

Limitations of Use:
Addyi is not indicated for the treatment of HSDD in postmenopausal women or in men.
Addyi is not indicated to "make sex better."

There was an "alcohol interaction study" with Addyi in twenty-three men and two premenopausal women. What was the alcohol interaction study? All twenty-five subjects, each of whom weighed 150 pounds, were administered Addyi 100 mg and the equivalent of two or four glasses of wine consumed over ten minutes when they woke up in the morning. The equivalent of two to four glasses of wine is two or four beers or two to four shots of 80 proof alcohol. A severe drop in blood pressure or fainting was seen in four out of twenty-three people who had the equivalent of two glasses of wine, and a couple of people needed medical help. Six out of the twenty-five subjects (25 percent) who were co-administered Addyi 100 mg and the equivalent of four glasses of wine over 10 minutes first thing in the morning experienced a blood pressure drop when standing from a sitting position. There were no events requiring someone needing help (therapeutic intervention) when Addyi or alcohol was administered alone. Therefore, a woman should not take Addyi, or Flibanserin, if she drinks alcohol or have liver disease or liver failure. Do not think that it is just the healthcare provider and the pharmacy that has to learn about the drug. Patients receiving the prescription must also sign a statement that says the following:

1. I understand I must not drink alcohol while taking Addyi (Flibanserin).

2. Drinking alcohol during treatment with Addyi has been shown to increase the risk of severe low blood pressure and fainting (loss of consciousness).

3. If I feel lightheaded or dizzy, I will lie down right away and seek medical help if these symptoms do not go away.

4. If I faint (lose consciousness), I will tell my healthcare provider as soon as possible.

5. I understand that I should only take Addyi at bedtime.

6. If I miss a dose, I will skip the missed dose. I will take my next dose the next day at bedtime.

The reader should be aware that the drug Wellbutrin (buproprion) has four times the fainting rate and twelve times the low blood pressure rate that is reported with Addyi. The FDA did not require a signed consent form prior to prescribing Wellbutrin.

Let me tell you what is positive about Addyi. This is the first drug ever approved for Hypoactive Sexual Desire Disorder (HSDD). This is a great moment in the field of sexual medicine. This is the first FDA-approved drug for women with decreased libido. Some women have biologic issues (as opposed to emotional issues) that cause low libido. Flibanserin, or Addyi, works by rebalancing key brain chemicals and is *not* a hormone. Women now have a choice of an approved drug just for them, not an off-label use of a drug approved for men. Just because there is a medical option does not mean that sexual counseling or sex therapy is not needed. It just gives healthcare providers another option to treat a problem that is very prevalent in women. Healthcare providers have enormous empathy and sympathy for women with low sexual desire. We are very excited to have a drug that will work in up to 60 percent of women with this problem. If you are a "responder" to the drug, you may have a doubling of your satisfying sexual events, up to a 53 percent increase in sexual desire (per the Female Sexual Function Index), and up to a 29 percent decrease in your distress about low libido.

When healthcare providers give you a new medication, you should be told about the benefits, side effects, and risks of the drug. We are not going to do anything different for this new medication for low libido. This drug will *not* make you hypersexual. This drug will not make sex "better." It will not make you a better lover. However, if you feel better and less distressed about your sexual experiences, your relationship with your intimate partner may improve significantly. Please be aware that there is no pill to fix a miserable relationship, an insensitive and uncaring partner, or anger that has accumulated in a marriage for many years. Both partners need to be very honest about why there is *not* a sexual relationship in a marriage.

45
Anger and Sleep Management

Very low-dose antidepressants or antianxiety medications help with the emotional changes of perimenopause and the menopausal transition. My favorite drug in the world to use for this is a low dose of Prozac or Paxil. If you read the medical journals and textbooks, you will see Effexor, Paxil, and Wellbutrin discussed for menopause. I personally think that the doses that physicians start people on are too high. Prozac, or fluoxetine, was the first SSRI (selective serotonin re-uptake inhibitor) that came on the market. It is cheap, and it is the only one approved for children and dogs. (Yes. Ask your veterinarian; they use it for depressed and anxious dogs.) It is also approved for PMS and works well for this. I give my patients a very low dose of Prozac for their menopausal symptoms and mood swings. A normal starting adult dose is 20 mg/day. A child's dose is 10 mg/day and a dog dose is 5 mg/day. I usually start my patients out on a 10 mg tablet that they break in half. If you think about it, they are not depressed but are overwhelmed with the changes that are happening to them. After about a month, I have them increase the dose to 10 mg/day if they are not any better. Most of the antidepressants that we use for menopausal symptoms are capsules, and they do not come in lower doses. I like to stay with this low dose of Prozac for several reasons. The 10 mg dosage is a tablet that can be cut in half, and this helps people wean off the drug when they are ready. It is hard to wean off a capsule unless you just take it less often—that is, every other day, then every third day, then every fourth day. Secondly, my patients do not usually need the higher dose, which is indicated for depression. Lastly, on the low dose, they do not have the side effects that can commonly occur with this class of drug. Some women have a terrible time sleeping. It is not just the night flushes, soaked t-shirt, and hot feet. It is an overwhelming feeling of anxiety that hits you right when you get in bed. You cannot shut your head off no matter how many sheep, butterflies, or pleasant thoughts are imagined. I frequently offer a low dose of Ambien for these patients. I think that 10 mg of Ambien is really too high a dose for most adults. I think that is why people do things in the middle of the night and do not remember what they did when they are on Ambien. The drug is working correctly; it is an hypnotic. I prescribe the 5 mg dose. I ask my patients to cut them in half. A dose of 2.5 mg of Ambien should shut your head off and help you sleep through the night flushes. A low dose of Xanax will also do the trick. I prescribe 0.25 mg of Xanax and have my patients cut them in half. It shuts their heads off at night so they can sleep through the misery of menopausal nights. I may sound like a big drug pusher to some readers. I am not. Each patient must be evaluated individually. I talk to them extensively about the risks of every drug that I prescribe for their symptoms. My patients are usually very apprehensive about starting any of these regimens, but when they walk out of my office, they are fully aware of my intention to put them on low (subclinical) doses.

46
THE ORGASM

What exactly is an orgasm? According to *Encyclopedia Britannica*, the orgasm is a physiological state of heightened sexual excitement and gratification that is followed by relaxation of sexual tensions and the body's muscles. Orgasm is marked by a feeling of sudden and intense pleasure, an abrupt increase in pulse rate and blood pressure, and spasms of the pelvic muscles that cause contractions of the lower vagina in the female and contractions of the urethra and ejaculation by the male. Orgasm can occur while a person is asleep and dreaming, as well as from sexual intercourse or masturbation. Generally, the differences between the human male and female orgasms are that the climax in the female can be physiologically interrupted more easily than can the male response. A male's orgasm is usually accompanied by ejaculation of semen. Both males and females experience momentary muscular contractions during the orgasm, but the female's effects are usually longer in duration. Since male responses are usually more rapidly induced, men achieve orgasm more consistently during intercourse than a woman. However, once a woman reaches orgasm, she remains sexually excited and, if stimulated, may experience several successive orgasms. In contrast, men are ordinarily unable to experience a second orgasm until after a variable waiting period. This is a very clinical definition.

Marie Nyswander Robinson MD, a Cornell-educated psychiatrist, devoted her New York City medical practice to the treatment of "frigidity" in women. Her book, *The Power of Sexual Surrender* (1958), reports that sexual satisfaction depends on self-surrender. Dr. Robinson's description of an orgasm is awesome. Orgasm is the physiological response, which brings sexual intercourse to its natural and beautiful termination. In the moment just preceding orgasm, muscular tension suddenly rises to the point where, if the sexual instinct were not in operation, it would become physically unendurable. The pelvic motions of the man and the movement of the penis back and forth within the vagina increase in speed and in intensity of thrust. The woman's pelvic movements also increase, and her whole body attempts with every move to heighten the exquisite sensations she is experiencing within her vagina. According to many women with whom I have discussed this experience, the greatest pleasure is caused by the sensation of fullness within the vagina and the pressure and friction upon its posterior surface. At the moment of greatest muscular tension, all sensations seem to take one further rise upward. The woman tenses beyond the point where, it seems, it would be impossible to maintain such tension for a moment longer. And indeed, it is not possible, and now her whole body suddenly plunges into a series of muscular spasms. These spasms take place within the vagina itself, shaking the body with waves of pleasure. They are felt simultaneously throughout the body: in the torso, face, arms, and legs, down to the very soles of the feet. These spasms, which shake the entire body and converge upon the vagina represent and define true orgasm. At this moment, the woman's head is thrown back and her pelvis tips upward in an attempt to obtain as much penetration from the penis as is possible. The spasms continue for several seconds in most women, though the time varies with each individual; and in some women, they may continue with decreasing intensity for a minute or even more. Many women can repeat this performance two or three times before their partner has his orgasm. The pathway, neurologically and psychologically, has been set for orgasm, and, if her partner continues, she can respond.

I have had women report that the last orgasm is sometimes more intense and satisfying than the first. If the woman is satisfied by her orgasmic experience, she will discharge the neurological and muscular tension developed in the sexual buildup. When satisfaction has been achieved, her strenuous movements cease and within a short period blood pressure, pulse, glandular secretion, muscular tension, and all the other gross physical changes, which characterizes sexual excitement, return to normal, or even to subnormal limits. There have been detailed studies made of the physical reactions of both men and women during intercourse. I think it is important to realize that in almost every detail, including orgasm, these reactions and the subjective experience of pleasure parallel each other in the sexes. The major differences are that the woman is slightly slower to respond at the outset than the man is, and the orgasm of the man is characterized by the ejaculation of sperm into the vagina. Full sexual satisfaction is followed by a state of utter calm. The body feels quiescent. Psychologically, the person feels completely satisfied, at peace with the world and all things in it. The woman, in particular, feels extremely loving toward the partner who has given her so much joy, such a transport of ecstasy. Often she wishes to hold him close for a while, to linger tenderly in the now subdued glow of their passion. As you can see from this description, an orgasm is a tremendous experience. There is no physiological or psychological experience that parallels the sweeping intensity or its excruciating pleasure. It is unique.

Wow. I don't think that I can top that description. Every time that I read that description, it makes me want to find my husband and have my own orgasm. Many women of all ages come into the office and want to ask questions about orgasms. After they get comfortable with our topic of conversation, many of them admit that they have never had an orgasm without clitoral stimulation; they think they are not normal. I tell them that not only is this normal for most women, but as women age, and especially after menopause, it takes even longer for women to achieve orgasm via clitoral stimulation. This is normal. It is just something we find hard to admit. In our society with entertainment outlets, cable television, the Internet, and movies, we are subjected to watching people having intercourse whether we want to or not. I suspect that watching women have these massive orgasms every time they have intercourse is what makes them feel inadequate if they do not respond the same way. I promise that what happens in your own bedroom is probably much more the normal response than what we see actors portraying. I have had so many women come in and admit that they are not sure they have ever had an orgasm. I believe them. I feel terrible for these women; my heart hurts for them so badly. The first thing a healthcare provider should do in this circumstance is make sure that the patient has not been sexually abused. This usually has a negative effect on her ability to relax in the bedroom. There may be some underlying issue that makes them unable to "let go" enough to reach an orgasm. I make sure that my patients know their own anatomy. If you are not sure where your clitoris is, then ask your OB/GYN. I promise, your doctor will not ridicule you or think badly of you if you do not know. We get this question all the time. I get this question in my office almost every day. As an OB/GYN, I have an advantage over psychotherapists and counselors in that I do not have to rely on diagrams; when the patient is undressed and I am doing a pelvic exam, I can give the patient a mirror. I can touch and point out the anatomy. An OB/GYN will not make you feel uncomfortable about not knowing your anatomy. If he or she does, then find another doctor. I do not know how to help women have an orgasm other than to show them their own anatomy so that they can pleasure themselves. I encourage reading books on the subject. I always recommend the purchase and use of a vibrator; I consider them an essential aid in these cases. I have always been told in my training that if a woman cannot stimulate herself to an orgasm by rubbing her clitoris, there is little chance that it will happen with intercourse. I suspect that this is true.

If the problem still exists and further work is needed, I suggest making an appointment with a reputable sex therapist. Occasionally a man will come into my office and somehow gets up the nerve to ask how to make his wife have an orgasm. I respect a man who has the guts to ask this; it must be hard to do. If he has come to this point, it is obvious the couple (or the woman) cannot talk about this together or are just too embarrassed. This is kind of an awkward moment for me. I really only know how I do it to myself and how I like it done, ya know? It's embarrassing.

Clearly, it is very hard for some men and women to talk about how to pleasure each other. If it were not, I would not have these conversations all the time. I only have my own body and my own response to rely on. I usually tell him to pay attention to her signals. If she is moaning in pleasure when you are rubbing up and down and moves your finger away when you are going side to side on the clitoris, well then, I would keep doing it up and down. I tell her to make sure that she gives him these signals. I also usually tell the man to go fast, but not hard. I always get a giant nod from the woman when I say that. One woman even cried and mouthed the word, "thank you", while nodding her head vigorously. I also say that, personally, moving your finger slowly up and down just pisses me off. Many women are appreciative of this comment. The other problem with this is that there are many of my patient's partners who know how I like to have an orgasm. I won't tell on you if you don't tell on me. Men must like to watch women give themselves an orgasm because my patients frequently tell me that their partner asks for this and it embarrasses them. I do not really have any specific advice for this. I am not in favor of doing something that makes you feel uncomfortable. However, at the same time, if you are married and that makes him happy, perhaps you could maybe do it for him occasionally. If you masturbate in front of him as an anniversary or birthday present, then you would only have to do it once a year. At least he could see how to do it correctly. Right?

47
VIBRATORS

I think that women should use vibrators regularly. Vibrators are wonderful. If you have never used a vibrator, you should consider "opening up" to the experience. When I recommend this in my office, I usually hear a response such as, "I'm a grandmother! I can't use one of those things!" I say, "Sure you can." At this point, I grab a vibrator, turn it on, and just place it in her lap. I will get a big smile from my patient who will usually comment, "Oh, I see. That's nice." Yes, it is. It is wonderful. It is wonderful even through the gown and her cover sheet. Can you imagine how much more wonderful it would be if it was directly on your clitoris?

Saying the word "vibrator" to a woman will usually bring up memories of bachelorette parties in our twenties. Someone always purchased a large penis-shaped vibrator and passed it around for all the girls at the party to play with and hold. Actually, the ones that I saw were frightening. They were abnormally large and came in a package with sexual sayings all over them. It was funny in the context of a bachelorette party with twenty girls screaming and laughing, but I doubt any of us left the party thinking that they would ever use one. The vibrators that I have in my office are slender, pretty, and coated in a soft silicone covering. The ones that I have are made by Pure Romance and Intimina. When I show them to my patients, I usually get a smile and a long, "Oh, very pretty!" When I walk my patients into my little retail store in the office where they can purchase these products, many of them are scared to walk through the door. When I motion them in, they say, "It's so pretty in here!" I am sure that they were expecting an adult toy-store atmosphere, but this is not pornography.

These products are used for personal massage, pleasure, and to help with stretching of the vagina. They are intimacy aids. I want you to use them to help keep your vagina in shape, stretched out, and functioning well. Vibrators come in all shapes and sizes. There are many websites where you can buy these products. They are also available in novelty stores. My patients always tell me that they are not surfing the web for these products and are not going to a novelty store to buy them. I used to purchase them for some women who asked me to get them for them until I found myself going to a novelty store all the time. I started having them available for sale in my office. It is a service for my patients. Many OB/GYNs are starting to have these available for purchase in their offices so that women do not have to be humiliated by walking into a novelty store. It is a safe place to shop for the patients, and they do not have to be embarrassed to have their cars in front of the store. In addition, you do not want to run into a neighbor, your Sunday school teacher, or someone you know. Vibrators can run on batteries or can be rechargeable. The rechargeable ones are usually more expensive. There are hundreds of sizes and shapes of vibrators. The cost can be from around ten dollars for a small battery operated one up to fifteen thousand and five hundred dollars for a 24-karat gold-plated vibrator. I kid you not. Clitoral vibrators are small oval-shaped vibrators that you can place strategically between the labia to get the vibration. The vibration is nice to feel even through your clothes. When I show a woman a vibrator, I usually turn it on high and place it on her lap. Usual response: "Oh! I see." It will stay in place if you wrap your labia around it. It takes most women a lot longer to have an orgasm after menopause. If a couple uses a vibrator as "foreplay," she is more likely to have an orgasm during intercourse. Most women can only have an orgasm with clitoral stimulation anyway. If you leave a small clitoral vibrator or bullet on the clitoris during intercourse, it might be just what you need. I have always thought to myself that the reason that God gave women the ability to have multiple orgasms is to make up for a lifetime of menstrual periods.

I think that if men would work on the woman and get her to have an orgasm first, then more women would be willing to have and enjoy the sexual act. A common complaint is that he ejaculates and then rolls over and falls asleep. Even if he says, "Are you okay?" he does not intend to fix the problem. Usually they say (as they are rolling over), "You're okay, right?" There are many women out there with blue balls syndrome. I always heard that in high school; the men would get excited and, being good Southern girls, we did not let them finish the job. Well, in this case, they got us back. For the rest of our lives, the men finish "the job" and then, we lay there all frustrated. I think that many women must get up to go urinate and finish off their orgasm in the bathroom. I think that all women should keep a vibrator hidden in the bathroom so that they can finish it off faster and get back to bed.

I recommend using a vibrator to many of my patients in my private practice. There are many reasons for my recommendation. An orgasm relieves a lot of stress, and women have a ton of stress. We are all working because you cannot make it with only one person in the family working. Women are the primary caregivers for their children, and with people living so long now, they are also the primary caregivers for their parents and in-laws. This is called the sandwich generation. Sometimes my patients tell me that a good orgasm (all by themselves) is all they have left. I understand. Once my patient gets over the embarrassment of buying a vibrator, they find it easier to talk about at the next visit. It also may cause problems that I did not intend her to have. For example, a woman might come in and say, "Doctor, I used a vibrator so much that my clitoris is numb. I'm scared that I broke the button." No worries; the nerve is just bruised a little. It will work again. I promise.

Clitoral vibrators come in multiple sizes and shapes. Sometimes they are referred to as "bullets." Vaginal vibrators are longer and are intended to place into your vagina. They have hundreds of shapes and can have a variety of additions to them to add to the pleasurable experience. There are combined clitoral and vaginal vibrators as well. These vaginal vibrators have a knob that sits on your clitoris at the same time. This way, you get stimulation to the vaginal and the clitoris simultaneously. You've got to try those! "G"-spot vibrators are shorter vaginal vibrators that reach up to stimulate a special area in the vagina. This area is about one inch inside your vagina. You can reach it by putting your middle finger into your vagina and lifting it up. There is a ridge of folds there that when stimulated give some women a very intense orgasm. Not all women have increased pleasure when this area is stimulated; every woman is made a little bit different. There are also vibrators that are combined "G"-spot and clitoral vibrators.

At this point I would like to get away from calling these products "vibrators." I am prescribing them as physical therapy for your vagina. In the following chapters I will discuss how this therapy can be implemented. I want to take the stigma of pornography off these products. It is not pornography. They are intimacy aids.

48
INTIMACY AIDS

What do you do with your intimacy aids ("vibrator" if you did not read the last chapter)? Well, the clitoral aid is placed on or to the side of your clitoris. You have to let go! Feel the vibrations throughout your whole pelvis, but concentrate on the sensation on your clitoris. You do not have to push down very hard unless you want to. Play with the different pressures and the different modes on your intimacy aid. Show your husband how you like it held there. Should he hold it steady or move it up and down or side to side? What do you like? Many of the aids have three to twelve different modes of vibration. For example, you may like constant intense vibration, little short pulses, or long intense pulses. Use this to have an orgasm by yourself to relieve stress or before intercourse to help get you in the mood. If your husband is interested, he can incorporate this into his foreplay; it will probably help him get aroused to see you have an orgasm first.

Joke: Why do so many women fake orgasm?
Answer: Because so many men fake foreplay.
(*Thank you to Michael Krychman, MD, for this joke.*)

Many of the clitoral aids or "bullets" are small enough to leave in place during intercourse. This will help bring you to orgasm during actual intercourse, and he will get some of the vibration. There are even "micro-bullets" that can be placed into the vagina. They can remain there during intercourse. A double micro-bullet is available so that you can place one of them on your clitoris and one inside your vagina. Lubricants can be placed on the vibrators if needed to help with insertion. Vaginal intimacy aids are placed into your vagina and are best used with your favorite lubricant. Some women like the vibration to penetrate the vaginal walls. You can manipulate your cervix with the aid and get some different muscle sensations.

Stretching Your Vagina
There are so many of my patients that were happy with many years of no sexual intercourse. They were happy to just be with their husbands and cuddle. Then,

after five or ten years, their husbands decided to ask the doctor for Viagra to help with an erection. It works. It can work too well. All of a sudden, they can have an erection and a good one. The woman has had many years of no activity in her vagina; it has decreased in width and in length. The folds in the vagina, which allow the vagina to maintain the accordion effect, are gone. Intercourse is painful. It is dry. It is not pleasant at all. She has done nothing during this time to keep her vagina in shape, because she thought that she did not ever have to have intercourse again. Many men leave their wives after thirty or forty years of marriage just because they cannot have intercourse. They go out and find a partner who can have intercourse. It is profoundly sad. I can help a woman get her vagina back (to a certain extent), but it is not going to be fast. It is surely not going to be as fast as Viagra works in men. What do I suggest? A good start is vaginal estrogen. I have already explained in an earlier chapter how this works. The tissues of the vagina will increase in thickness, the blood flow will increase, and the lubrication glands will start working again. If it took five or ten years to atrophy, it is going to take a while to improve. Hang in there. I want my patients to use the vibrator as physical therapy. A vibrator will help to get the blood flowing to the area again.

There are two reasons to use a vibrator: pleasure and physical therapy. I encourage women to use a vibrator for pleasure. It is wonderful. Knock yourself out. In the office, however, I am talking about using the vibrator to get the blood flowing to the area and to stretch the vagina back out to its previous width and length. I have my patients put some estrogen cream on the vibrator to use it as a lubricant. She can put it in the vagina slowly, with the vibrator on full vibration, just watch TV or a movie, and leave it in there for fifteen to thirty minutes. If the vagina has decreased in width and length, then she can start with a small, thin vibrator and slowly (under her own pressure) stretch out the vagina. It will stretch back out. How do I know this? Well, there are women born without vaginas. This is called the Mayer-Rokitansky-Kuster-Hauser syndrome. Most of us just call it Rokitansky syndrome. It is a congenital anomaly (it happens during growth in the womb) where the patient has the outside female parts but not the inside female parts. It occurs in about one in five thousand to one in ten thousand females. They cannot have a baby, but if they had a vagina, they could have intercourse. It is very sad. Otherwise, you would never know that anything is wrong with them. They have ovaries, so they look like any other woman except for not having a vagina or a functioning uterus. Well, surgeons tried to make for them vaginas by boring a hole into that area of the body (where the vagina should have been) and then using skin grafts to make the skin of the vagina. It sometimes works. Then physicians realized that the tissue in this area had the ability to stretch. Think about the women in Africa that put the rings around their necks and stretch their necks to great lengths. Although this takes many years, and they start it when they are young, it is the same principle.

Physicians designed a stand with a girl's bicycle seat on it. The girl screws a peg onto the bicycle seat and sits on it for about an hour a day. They increase the size of the peg every couple of weeks until the peg is the size of a normal vagina. If she works hard at this and does it every day, the girl can have a normal-sized vagina in about six months to a year. These women have normal sex lives; they just cannot have a baby, as there is no uterus at the top of the vagina. I have several patients that have this syndrome. They come in for annual examinations and Pap smears just like women without this syndrome. A pelvic exam is done to feel their ovaries inside and make sure that there are no masses. I can remember one patient in particular. She came in for her annual exam and I could not find her vagina. I pushed the sheet down to look at her, and said, "You really have not been a busy girl down here." She said, "Has my vagina shrunk up? Never mind, I know it has. We have been so busy building a new house and helping our kids with the grandchildren, we haven't been having intercourse much." Women with this syndrome need either to have intercourse regularly or put in a dilator regularly to keep the vagina from shrinking up. However, they can get it back with some work. When she came in the next year, her vagina was long and wide. I shoved the sheet down again, and said, "Oh my goodness! What a difference!" She said, "I know. After I left last year, I told my husband that there was hardly a hole anymore. We made a New Years' resolution to make sure that never happens again. We have been very busy." My point in telling you this story is that you already have the vagina. You just have to keep it stretched out in some way. You are already way ahead of women with Rokitansky syndrome! You already have the hole. Stretch it out! Get the vibrator and put it on high vibration. Watch TV and get it in shape. It is not going to happen overnight, but it will happen. When you are in bed at night, put your intimacy aid (vibrator) in your vagina and keep it at high vibration. The vibration is going to help with the blood flow to the area. You can start with a small, thin aid and then gradually increase to one that is more appropriate for the size of your husband's penis. When you are stretching your vagina yourself, you are controlling the pressure, not your husband; and you can do it at your own pace. This way you can stretch your vagina without the anxiety that comes with the fear of pain from the perhaps quick insertion or thrusting of the penis. You are controlling everything. You can place vaginal cream on the intimacy aid to use as a lubricant and to stimulate the estrogen receptors. If you start stretching your vagina daily, you will see improvement in the diameter just like going to the gym everyday will increase the size of your muscles. If you also squeeze the muscles in your vagina (Kegel exercises) around the intimacy aid, you will help these muscles also. Almost all of us watch television for an hour or so at night or read a book prior to going to bed. Put your vibrator in during this time and kill two birds with one stone.

49
AROUSAL OILS, MOISTURIZERS, AND LUBRICANTS

Arousal oils

Arousal oils are a variety of combinations of herbs, oils, and sometimes cinnamon and/or menthol that are mixed together to stimulate the clitoris and surrounding labia. This is the erectile tissue in the female that corresponds to the erectile tissue in the male—the penis. Arousal oils make the whole area warm and tingly. This makes the blood rush into the labia (remember, they have a huge blood supply and are made up of erectile tissue) and helps your clitoris become stimulated. Arousal oils may also give a "cooling" sensation to the area. This works very nicely and totally is a matter of preference. Some women like warming oils and some like cooling oils. That is why there is chocolate and vanilla. Two very common arousal oils are: ON (Sensuva) and Zestra. They can be ordered on the internet.

Moisturizers

Is there a difference between vaginal moisturizers and vaginal lubricants? Yes! We probably all have a moisturizing regimen when we get out of the shower. You put moisturizer on your face before you apply makeup. You would not consider going out of the house without moisturizer on your hands. You probably have some in your car and in your desk at work. In fact, you probably put moisturizer on your hands throughout the day, especially in the winter when they dry out. So be that nice to your vagina! She is drying out! Take care of her!

Several vaginal moisturizers can be used just as if you would use regular moisturizers on your face, hands, or body. These safe, non-hormonal products work well for mild symptoms. They are different from using lubricants for vaginal intercourse. I am talking about routine moisturizing. They are intended for use multiple times per week or even daily. You would not consider putting lotion on your hands just once a week and expect the skin on your hands to be soft and pliable. Most women put lotion on their hands many times per day. Granted, the skin of your hands is exposed to soap and air all the time, but you get the picture. Only you can take care of your vagina. Some examples of these products are Just Like Me (Pure Romance), Replens, Me Again, Hyalo-gyn, Luvena, coconut oil, and vegetable oil. In my office, I sell vaginal syringes so that this is easier to get the oil up in there. You do not need much, just a little dip on your finger, put it up in there, and coat the walls. Keep them soft and pliable. I want to change the morning regimen for women everywhere. Get out of the shower and dry off. But at this point, if you are truly menopausal, you have had a major hot flash and are soaked with sweat. If so, get back in the shower and rinse off. Repeat until you are so pissed off that you cannot rinse off anymore. Put your favorite moisturizer on your body. Put a little bit of your favorite vaginal moisturizer on your finger (or in your vaginal syringe) and take care of your vagina. Wash your hands and then you can moisturize your face and proceed with your makeup. Five seconds of your time spent on your vagina is all it will take to keep her moisturized, happy, and healthy.

Lubricants

If you are forty-five or older, you probably need a lubricant for intercourse. It has nothing to do with how much you love your partner. It has nothing to do with how much you enjoy lovemaking. It has nothing to do with him "turning you on." It has nothing to do with whether you think he is still hot. The ovaries are failing! The vagina does not have the estrogen stimulation that it used to, and the lubrication glands do not work as well. You have to use something to allow the penis to slide in and out of there. Otherwise, it is like swiping a cotton ball over sandspurs. It is dry; the tissue will "catch" and may even bleed from the friction. The vagina itself can take a lot of abuse, but the skin of the vagina is fragile like butterfly wings after menopause.

There are four types of lubricants: water-based, silicone, oil-based, and hybrid

Water based lubricants are the most popular and can be used safely with sex toys, latex condoms, diaphragms, and sponges. They are probably the best to use for people who have sensitive skin or are prone to allergic reactions. They are very easy to clean up and they dry up easily. They do not stain sheets and are easily removed in the washing machine. Some have sugar, flavors, and/or glycerin in them. They can be reactivated by adding a little water.

Silicone-based lubricants do not break down in water so they last a long time and you do not need to reapply as often. They work great in the tub, shower, hot tub, and pool. Many people cannot have intercourse except in water because of arthritis or pain in joints. It helps them get into positions that normally they could not maintain due to pain or low flexibility. The problem is that is it very slippery and can cause you to fall in the shower or on a tile floor. Silicone sex toys cannot be combined with silicone lubricant, because the toy may be ruined. They cannot be used on latex condoms or diaphragms because the material will break down and allow sperm to get into the uterus. Silicone is difficult to wash off of beds and may stain the sheets. They are usually more expensive than water-based lubricants.

Oil-based lubricants are thick and have good lubrication, but they can cause latex condoms to tear. Oil-based lubricants include Vaseline, vegetable oils, coconut oil, and Vitamin E oil. They cannot be used with rubber toys because they can ruin them. They may be good for people in monogamous relationships who do not have to worry about pregnancy concerns. They are a little messy (as you can imagine), and clothing needs to be washed in the washing machine.

Hybrid lubricants have a combination of water-based lubricant and silicone. They can be slippery, but not enough to take away sensation. They can be used as moisturizers because they hydrate and keep moisture in the skin. They cannot be used with silicone toys. Many of them can be used with latex and rubber, so check the label.

There are many different lubricants for intercourse. Some are awesome and fun. My favorite is Sensations Hot Buttered Rum by Pure Romance. There are many different types of lubricants: warming lubricants, cooling lubricants, tingling lubricants, his and her lubricants, homemade lubricants, organic lubricants, lubricants with lots of preservatives, and flavored lubricants. Why don't you know about all these? Because we all buy lubricants the same way. A woman goes to the grocery store and hovers around the lubricant aisle. When she sees that no one is in the aisle, she runs up to the lubricants, throws the one that she usually gets into the basket, and hurries down to the toilet paper area. She puts some toilet paper and tissues on top of the lubricant so that no one sees it. When she gets to the checkout line, she prays that it has a barcode on it and the young bagger will not have to go get a price check. When she gets home, she quickly takes the lubricant out of the box and shoves the box in the bottom of the trashcan so that the kids do not see it. She hides the bottle in the bedroom. She now relaxes a bit and puts away the groceries. Does this sound familiar? She never reads the label, the ingredients, the calories (you never know, it could have calories), or the cholesterol and fat content. Have you ever seen anyone comparing labels to lubricants in any store? No. Have you ever seen anyone asking the employees which one is the most popular? No. It is all a big secret that we all use it.

I tell my patients to try vegetable oil. They look at me funny at first, but I explain it in the following way. Think about how soft and pliable your hands would be if you applied vegetable oil on them instead of lotion. The oil would get all over everything that you touched, but they would feel good. I do not mean that you have to have vegetable oil dripping out of your vagina, but if you just dipped your finger in it and coated the walls of your vagina, they would be soft and pliable. There is nothing special about vegetable oil; you could use canola, olive, coconut, or peanut oil. I have many patients that use coconut oil. These may be messy and you may need a pad, but it sticks around and works very well.

I have a great story about vegetable oil. I told this woman at her annual exam how vegetable oil may help with the pain of intercourse. She went home and told her husband, and it obviously worked well for them. How did I know this? Well, the next year at her annual exam, I opened the door and greeted her in my usual fashion. It was just when I was giving her a hug that I noticed her husband in the room. He had a big smile on his face and said, "I have been waiting a year to come and see you with my wife. I couldn't wait to get here." I looked at her and she rolled her eyes. She said, "That's right, he has been waiting a year for this. I hear it all the time. He tells me that he can't wait to see Dr. Pam to tell her." I looked at him. "Tell me what?" He said, "You told my wife that we should try vegetable oil as a lubricant for intercourse."

I said, "Yes, I have lots of couples who love it." He said, "Well, we love it; I love it. It is the best lubricant in the whole world!" I said, "I'm glad that I could help." He said, "The best part is that I call it frying chicken." I looked at my patient, and she rolled her eyes again. He said, "Whenever I want to make love, I tell her that we need to fry some chicken. I love frying chicken. Frying chicken is the best part of my day! I have been waiting a whole year to tell you that." He laughed hysterically, got up, and left. I looked at her. She rolled her eyes and said, "He's been waiting for a year to tell you that. He even wanted me to come in early until he found out that the insurance wouldn't pay to come early." I'm glad that I could help.

These products help with dryness and pliability, but do not stop the process of atrophy and thinning. The only thing that you can do to stop the process is replacing the estrogen in this area so that those estrogen receptors in your vagina and surrounding areas are working. You need to turn those receptors "on."

50
GIVE YOURSELF PERMISSION TO LET GO!

One thing that my patients worry about is what their pastor, priest, rabbi, or minister thinks about them using intimacy aids. Not how the spiritual adviser feels personally, but women feel that they are being immoral if they use vibrators. I think that there is nothing further from the truth. Those of us that were brought up with biblical teachings are well aware that the Bible warns us against immorality. We hear about the sinful nature of the works of the flesh, fornication, and adultery. We are told to put to death any earthly desires such as sexual immorality, impurity, lust, and evil desires. However, from a biblical standpoint marriage is sacred and supported. The Song of Solomon is a wedding song that every married couple should read; it is a celebration of the love between a married man and woman. The book promotes loyalty, beauty, and sexuality in the marriage. It is also a book that speaks to unmarried women. The daughters of Jerusalem are encouraged to wait for sexual intimacy until after marriage. The book portrays the joys of love in courtship and marriage, and the rightful place of physical love in marriage is clearly established and honored. The Song of Solomon is God's provision to sustain loving marriages and renew loveless ones. Consider these passages: 4:1–16 and 5:1 This passage has Solomon talking (singing) to his bride on the night of their consummation of the marriage. He is gazing upon her and taking in her beauty one body part at a time. Then Solomon asks that his bride gather her scattered thoughts, allay her fears, and give herself solely to him. The term "sister" is an affectionate name for one's wife.

1 "How beautiful you are my darling,
   How beautiful you are!
   Your eyes are like doves behind your veil;
   Your hair is like a flock of goats
   That have descended from Mount Gilead.
2 Your teeth are like a flock of newly shorn ewes
   Which have come up from their washing,
   All of which bear twins,
   And not one among them has lost her young.

3   Your lips are like a scarlet thread,
    And your mouth is lovely.
    Your temples are like a slice of a pomegranate
    Behind your veil.
4   Your neck is like the tower of David,
    Built with rows of stones
        On which are hung a thousand shields,
    All the round shields of the mighty men.
5   Your two breasts are like two fawns,
    Twins of a gazelle
    Which feed among the lilies.
6   Until the cool of the day
    When the shadows flee away,
    I will go my way to the mountain of myrrh
    And to the hill of frankincense.
7   You are altogether beautiful, my darling,
    And there is no blemish in you.
8   Come with me from Lebanon, my bride,
    May you come with me from Lebanon.
    Journey down from the summit of Amana,
    From the summit of Senir and Hermon,
    From the dens of lions,
    From the mountains of leopards.
9   You have made my heart beat faster, my sister, my bride;
    You have made my heart beat faster with a single glance of your eyes,
    With a single strand of your necklace.
10 How beautiful is your love, my sister, my bride!
    How much better is your love than wine, and the fragrance of your oils
    Than all kinds of spices!
11 Your lips, my bride, drip honey;
    Honey and mild are under your tongue,
    And the fragrance of your garments is like the
    fragrance of Lebanon.

Solomon expresses his desire to consummate his marriage using the imagery of coming into a garden:

12 A garden locked is my sister, my bride,
   A rock garden locked, a spring sealed up.

13 Your shoots are an orchard of pomegranates
   With choice fruits, henna with nard plants.

14 Ntard and saffron, calamus and cinnamon,
   With all the trees of frankincense, myrhh and aloes,
   along with all the finest spices.

15 You are a garden spring,
   A well of fresh water,
   And streams flowing from Lebanon."

The bride then says the following to Solomon. She invites him into her garden using the same imagery.

16 "Awake, O north wind,
   And come, wind of the south;
   Make my garden breathe out fragrance,
   Let its spices be wafted abroad.
   May my beloved come to his garden
   And eat its choice fruits!"

Solomon then speaks to his bride about the consummation of the marriage. Solomon 5:1

   "I have come into my garden, my sister, my bride;
   I have gathered my myrrh along with my balsam.
   I have eaten my honeycomb and my honey;
   I have drunk my wine and my milk.

Then God replies to the couple.

   "Eat, friends;
   Drink and imbibe deeply, O lovers."

God intended us to be sexual and sensual in marriage. There are many books available on this subject if you don't feel comfortable talking to your pastor, priest, rabbi, or minister.

Once my patients understand that they have to keep their vaginas active in order to have intercourse for many years after menopause, they have a moment of anxiety. They laugh a little and usually say, "I can't do that! I'm a grandmother!" In my opinion it is fine for a grandmother or even a great-grandmother to have sex. The majority of women in menopause that come to see me for help and advice are very excited to hear what I have to say. At first they feel embarrassed that I talk about the parts of the male and female body so easily, but then this ease of speaking transfers to them quickly. I have a short period during their visit to give them as much information as possible. I want to give them all the information in this book, but obviously it cannot be done in one visit. In many cases I spend several minutes of the visit giving women permission to care for their vaginas as they have never cared for them before. It is not terribly different from a mother giving her child permission to go somewhere. Children need permission to go somewhere so that their mother will know where they are and that what they are doing is safe and acceptable.

In years past, women have never really had to take care of their vaginas. In 1900 the life expectancy for women was fifty years of age, so women did not even live long enough to go through menopause. In 1950 the life expectancy was seventy-one years of age; however, women suffered menopausal symptoms in silence as this was not the topic of normal conversation. Physicians were learning about estrogen and how it could help with their symptoms. In 2010 the average life expectancy at birth for women was eighty-one years. Women and men now are vibrant and physically active into their seventies and even into their eighties.

In 1998 the definition of "activity" changed for men and especially for women. Viagra, a drug for erectile dysfunction in men, was released. Men who were older had several medical problems, or who were on certain medications may have had difficulty maintaining an erection. If they took Viagra, these problems completely disappeared. Many women were living with their husbands for years without sexual activity. All of a sudden (really, within thirty minutes), their husbands could maintain an erection. Over the last sixteen years, more and more men have become comfortable talking with their physicians about erectile dysfunction.

In the opinion of this gynecologist, Viagra has been one of the worst things to happen to long-term marriages. This is not at all meant to be derogatory to the makers of Viagra. The drug probably works better than any other new drug that has come out in the last twenty years. There are now two other drugs for erectile dysfunction: Levitra and Cialis. They all work very well.

The American public has been inundated with advertisements for these drugs, and now young children are asking about erectile dysfunction because they see it on TV. Many of them even know what it means! The problems that post-menopausal women have in the area of sexual dysfunction are just now being discussed. Sixteen years after Viagra was released we are just now seeing television commercials about vaginal dryness! Why did it take so long? If you think about it, women married to men who have taken Viagra for the last sixteen years have been done a great disservice. They have suffered in silence, and many marriages have ended because women have been unable to have intercourse because of pain and dryness. It is time for women to take care of their vaginas! You have to use it or lose it.

The bottom line is that you have to keep your vagina active and healthy. This physician (me) knows this and is giving you permission to do the physical therapy that is needed to keep it in shape. It is not disgusting or degrading, and it is not pornography. We do not have a pill to keep this area of the body functioning well, and until we do, you have to take the preceding chapters in this book to heart. Women have to do some things that they never dreamed of doing.

The Five Types of Women

51
WOMEN WHO DO NOT HAVE A PARTNER AND ARE VERY GLAD NOT TO HAVE A PARTNER

There are some women who have been hurt very badly, by either abuse or divorce, who are very happy to be alone and in charge of their own lives again. They may be a little lonely at times but are extremely content. They are just very happy to be alone and safe. They do much better if they have children and grandchildren to fill their lives with love. Those who do not have children are usually very content with their beloved dog or cat that reciprocates their unconditional love. They have girlfriends who are of a similar mindset, and go on trips together, go to bingo, play cards, sip their wine and fancy drinks at night, and are extremely happy to go home alone. I do not worry about these women.

They are in a good place and are extremely content. They do not complain. I think that everyone in this category should consider an intimacy aid. As I have said before an, orgasm relieves stress and the release of tension can help you sleep better. There is always the possibility that they will meet someone later in life, and they should keep their vaginas stretched out.

52

WOMEN WHO WANT SEX AND DON'T HAVE A PARTNER

There are so many women out there over fifty who are craving a relationship. When I ask if they are sexually active they become tearful and say, "I only wish I was." They would welcome a sexual partner, but they really want to share their lives with someone. The sexual relationship is a big part of any relationship. They want a companion with whom to share their happiness and sorrows, joys and disappointments. They are craving romance. I wish some of the men their age would consider a woman who is not ten to fifteen years younger than they are. Almost every one of them says that even when they meet someone, the men tell them that they are looking for someone younger. Now, many women who are over fifty are very frightened to have a relationship. They are very frightened of sexually transmitted diseases. They do not understand the sexual promiscuity of the younger generation, and they do not want to feel pressured to move into a sexual relationship quickly. Most of them are divorced and want to take things slowly. One woman said to me, "I'm single; I'm too scared to have a relationship. These days, you have to boil someone to sleep with them." However, they constantly hint that they would welcome a partner. They are lonely. I encourage women in this category to keep their vaginas in good shape. There are men out there and many find someone after a couple of years. I encourage them to use a vibrator to keep the blood flowing to the vaginal tissues and to use vaginal estrogen to keep the folds in good condition. As I explained earlier, if you don't use it, you lose it. It is very hard to get your vagina back in shape for intercourse after years of atrophy. I encourage my patients to learn to enjoy an intimacy aid (vibrator). Many women out there are using things around the house to stimulate themselves. We have wonderful intimacy aids that are so much better. I have a perfect example. A patient came into the office with the complaint of irritation to her genitals, and she told me that she was in terrible pain. She was walking cautiously to get up on the exam table, and while I was helping her up there, I was thinking about all of the possibilities that could make this happen. I helped her lie down and said, "Let me see what you're talking about because now you have me worried." Well, I sat down between her legs, lifted the sheet back, and gasped in horror. She looked like she had had a fight with a cat, an angry cat. I stood up and walked over to the top of the table, held her hand and said, "What happened?" I really was frightened that someone had been abusive. The scratches were terrible. She sheepishly held her head down and said, "I have been masturbating." I replied, "With what?" She said, "A hair brush." I did not understand right away, and then it hit me. I said, "Turn it over. The handle would be better than the bristles." I explained to her that there were devices to use for masturbating that were wonderful.

53

WOMEN WHO WANT SEX AND HAVE A PARTNER WHO DOESN'T (OR CAN'T)

This is an extremely sad situation for both partners. This usually occurs when a man has a problem maintaining an erection or has had some type of surgery or medical problem that prevents him from having intercourse. This may be prostate surgery, diabetes, hypertension, radiation therapy, stroke, or some type of cancer, which has caused damage to the nerves or blood vessels to the penis, or, who knows why? Unfortunately, I think that both husband and wife would like to try to remedy the situation, but they cannot talk about it. Men put a lot of their self-worth into their ability to have sex. I believe that they feel it is part of their job to take care of and provide for their families, and somehow, having sex is part of how they feel manly. When something happens and they get sick and "things" do not work, their manhood is threatened. They do not feel that they are holding up their part of the bargain for the marriage. Do I have any data to support this? Yes. I wish that they knew that their wives do not feel that way. They do not see them as any less of a man. The women, however, still want the romance even if there is no sexual intercourse involved. They want their husbands to show that they love them in other ways. They still want the flowers, the wine with dinner, the walks around the block holding hands, and the snuggling. They all have the same complaints. Most of the time, I hear the words "He can't do it, so I am being punished, too. He could take care of me [give her an orgasm], but he chooses not to." It may sound like I am getting in a healthy dose of male bashing, but I hear it too often for it not to be true. These patients come in and feel frustrated. They say that they have carpal tunnel syndrome from doing hand jobs all the time. Their husbands cannot keep an erection long enough to penetrate the vagina, but they can have an orgasm if their wives work hard enough. The problem is that there is no quid pro quo. There is no reciprocity.

Many of my patients report that even though they have suggested that their husbands talk to their doctors about Viagra, they refuse to do so. They are too embarrassed, or humiliated, or do not want to admit that they have a problem. You may not believe this, but many men are too scared to take the drug. They are frightened of the side effects. How wonderful it would be if their husbands would look at them lovingly when they get in bed, and say, "Can I take care of you?" As I said earlier, most women cannot have an orgasm without clitoral stimulation, especially after menopause. Most of these women would be in absolute heaven if their husbands brought them to orgasm. I am sure that there are many men who do take care of their wives' sexual needs. Obviously, these women are not the ones complaining to their doctor (especially me) about the problem. I assume that they are happy. Doctors, too, only hear about the squeaky wheel. The other thing that women feel upset about is if they are constantly asked to perform oral sex because their husband cannot maintain an erection long enough for vaginal penetration. Again, it is fine if there is some reciprocity. These patients are just tired of always being the giver. So, what can these women do? Well, there are some things to help. For oral sex, there are flavored, warming lubricants. The warming part may help blood flow into the penis; the flavored just tastes better. You already know that condoms even come in a whiskey flavor. There are lubricants from Pure Romance that come in hot buttered rum, cosmopolitan, berry, and several other flavors.

Pure Romance also has products for men that may help. For instance, one product is like a "fake vagina." Men can put this on their penis (with plenty of lubricant) and their wives can give them a hand job, which works much better. Sometimes, women come in and complain that they are getting carpal tunnel syndrome from having to work so hard at this. This can help. There are also soft rings that they can put at the base of their penises that hold the blood in so that it can stay erect. They are called cock rings. They work very well in many men. If this is not an option in your marriage, then keep a vibrator in the bathroom. Take care of yourself quickly, and get back to bed. We have busy lives. You have to start over again tomorrow.

54

WOMEN WHO DON'T WANT SEX AND WHO ARE WITH MEN WHO DO

This is the most common category of women. This category is also profoundly sad for both husband and wife. Something happens when women go through menopause. There is a profound drop in libido. Women come into the office and are so upset that they have no libido. They cry. They want to have sex and they know that their husbands are upset about not having it. They wish they had some desire. One patient who was tired of having intercourse said to me, "I'm married; there is no time off for good behavior and no early parole." They are aware that their lack of libido is affecting their marriage, but they cannot fix it. Why is this? I can talk all day long about the lack of estrogen and testosterone. However, what causes this profound drop in libido? It is multifactorial. Anger and resentment play a major role here whether we are willing to admit it or not. We cannot forget about all the things that have pissed us off for the last several years. We remember that we had no help with the kids, diaper changes, meal preparation, housework, and everything else. We remember the times that we were criticized and made to feel worthless. You have to admit the anger and let it go. Don't use sex as a way to keep power over someone. Don't use sex as a weapon.

I personally remember one specific incident in my life. My husband was also a physician. He had come home early one day. He was relaxing on the couch and watching sports on the television. He did not look at me and put his hand up in the air as if he were holding a beer can and said, "Beer." Although annoyed and tired from a long day at work, I went back down to the garage to get a beer out of his beer fridge. I popped the beer and put it in his hand. He never looked at me and took a long swig. Still watching television, he said, "What's for dinner?" I said, "I don't know, what did you make?" He became very angry and said, "That's not funny." He was right; it wasn't funny. However, I sucked it up and made dinner. Obviously he did not get me naked that night. Three days later I came home to the dishwasher empty and the laundry started. He got it. But when I look back on it, I was wrong. I should have talked to him about my anger after we had both calmed down. I used sex as a weapon. It is wrong. The problem is that I still remember that incident from over ten years ago. It still pisses me off. I have to let it go. It is hard to do. That was a dumb little argument, and I am almost embarrassed to share it with the reader; however, it is a thousand little arguments that build up over the years that make us resent someone. We all have to start over, if possible, with a clean slate. We have to let all those little stupid arguments not build up. We cannot use (withholding) sex as a weapon when it should be a way to forget about those little arguments and show our love for each other.

I also think that a major contributor is the weight gain that happens around the time of menopause. Women are ashamed and embarrassed by what has happened to their body. They have low self-esteem because of their weight. It is hard to want to have sex when you do not feel sexy.

What can I do in these circumstances to help my patient? If you are willing to take the risk, I can prescribe you estrogen and testosterone. I can inform you of the products that may help. What can you do? If I said, "You can lose weight," I would alienate and piss off about fifty million women. It is so much harder to lose weight after menopause. On the other hand, if a patient got down to a size ten or twelve again, she would love the way she looked. She would get some of her self-esteem back. When we have self-esteem, we have self-confidence. Everyone notices when you have self-confidence. Aside from losing weight make yourself feel pretty. I can remember when my husband was very ill, and I was coming home from work exhausted. I went into the bedroom, took off my work clothes, and put on sweat pants, slippers, and an old t-shirt. When I walked out of the bedroom, my husband looked at me and said, "Oh, that's attractive." What? I was working, had two young children, was taking care of the house and a very sick husband who had IV fluids, a feeding tube, and could barely walk. Was he kidding? Probably, but it made me feel ugly. I wish I did not remember that. For the men out there reading this, we cannot remember where we left the keys or to bring milk home, but we remember every word of every conversation when our feelings are hurt. When you want to have sex, we remember that you implied that we did not look nice. I think that the key to having a better attitude about having sex is to know in advance that your husband wants to have sex. Your behavior will change if you know. For instance, say you fall into bed at night after a long day and finally get very comfortable and snuggled into your favorite position. Then, you get a little shake. Your husband says, "Hey, what do you think?" Oh My God. Are you kidding? What are you really thinking? I can tell you what I am thinking. When I would get that little shake, I really am thinking, "Oh no! I'm not prepared! I didn't take a shower!

What if I smell? My legs aren't shaved, I have been running around all day, and I would have brushed my teeth for thirty more seconds. I would have used mouthwash. I would have put something cute on, not my old t-shirt and your boxer shorts. And, you thought that I was ugly nine weeks ago."

What if, at the beginning of the day, your husband said, "I really would like to make love to you tonight." Wow. What would you do differently? You would come straight home after work and not go to the grocery store. I hope that you would leave the housework and laundry alone. If you have children at home you will get takeout for them instead of making dinner. If you do not have kids at home you may make a light dinner and have a glass of wine and some candles. You will probably take a shower, shave, put on lotion, put on perfume, and wear something pretty. Put on a negligee that you had shoved in the back of your pajama drawer. When you feel good about yourself, it will show. Imagine if you had two days' notice that he wanted to make love; you may even get butterflies in your stomach when you see him. Remember when you were dating? You got prettied up and felt good about yourself. We looked forward to the weekend, and that excitement helped with our desire. Go to a lingerie store and get something sexy. Perhaps you could read some erotica. If you have not read *Fifty Shades of Grey*, you should consider it. I do not personally like the S&M/dominatrix stuff. However, it is a good book to read before you plan to have sex. If you do finish the four-book series, you will realize that, overall, it is a love story. Women do like a good love story.

I was on a plane when I was reading the first book of the series. I sat down next to this young woman, and we said hello to each other. We made a little small talk. I was a little anxious to get back to my book (which was open in my hands) when she said, "I notice that you are reading *Fifty Shades of Grey*." I said, "Yes, I am." (Oh no! I do not want to get into a conversation about this book on a plane.) As she took a Kindle out of her bag, she said, "Actually, I am reading it, too. Do you mind if we don't talk anymore?" I laughed and said, "I would love to not talk to you." We read the entire three hours of the trip. Neither one of us got up to go to the bathroom, accepted a drink, or had snacks. When we got to our destination, she said, "It was so nice not talking to you." I said, "I agree completely." It is very difficult to read that book and not get aroused. When we stood up, she realized that my husband was sitting across the aisle from me. She said, "Oh my goodness, if I had known that that was your husband, I would have traded seats with him. I said, "It was probably better for everyone on this plane that he was not sitting next to me. I think that maybe you can be arrested for doing certain things in public. She said, "You know, you are probably right."

There were four men planning on going on a golf trip. They had been planning this trip for a while, and it was time to shore up the details of the trip. They met at the golf club to discuss the final details. One of the men came in and was obviously very upset. He said, "Guys, I am so very sorry; my wife and I got into an argument, and she will not let me go on the trip." They were disappointed, but figured that they would get someone to make up their foursome at the golf resort. A month later, the three men that went on the trip walked into the golf resort, and there, sitting at the bar, was their friend who thought that he could not go on the trip. He had a couple of shots of whiskey waiting for them, and they all had a toast to a promise of a great week of golf. One of the men said, "By the way, how did you get your wife to let you come with us this week?" He looked at them mischievously and said, "Since I saw you last month, my wife read the book *Fifty Shades of Grey*. I came home from work yesterday and she had on a negligee, smelled great, and had candles all over the bedroom. She took out a pair of handcuffs, and had me cuff her to the bedposts. She then told me that I could do anything that I wanted. I told her that I wanted to go on this golfing trip."

There are other things that you can do to get in the mood. Masturbate prior to getting into bed with or without a vibrator to get the vagina lubricated. If he is interested, and neither of you are upset by it, have him use a vibrator on you to have an orgasm first and then have intercourse. No matter what you read in *Cosmopolitan*, most women, especially postmenopausal women, have to stimulate the clitoris to have an orgasm. This is an excellent time to put on an arousal oil to get a good flow of blood to the labia, clitoris, and vagina. Then use a clitoral vibrator on the clitoris.

Just like in men, there are medications that can decrease your libido. Elevated blood pressure can affect the small blood vessels in your genital region and, unfortunately, blood pressure medication can affect sexual response. Some antacid medications can affect libido as well. There is nothing worse for libido than chronic depression. If you cannot even find a reason to get out of bed in the morning, then having sex is probably not going to be on the list either. Unfortunately, the medication that is the worst for libido is an antidepressant. Any of the selective serotonin re-uptake inhibitors (SSRIs) or the serotonin-norepinephrine re-uptake inhibitors (SNRIs) can make it difficult to have an orgasm in men and women.

These are drugs like Prozac, Zoloft, Paxil, and Lexapro. Many of the other types of antidepressants cause a decrease in libido also. Tricyclic antidepressants, antipsychotics, and antianxiety medications all affect libido. How frustrating is this? You finally get out of bed and treat your depression, your anxiety, or your illness and then you cannot reach an orgasm because of the medication that you were put on to treat the illness! How unfair is this? Ugh! You can start to feel good, but just never reach the goal. The ability to have an orgasm comes back when you get off the medication, but it is extremely frustrating. I have many women just stop their antidepressants when this happens. They tell me that they would rather be depressed than lose the ability to have an orgasm. I really would rather that they wean down to a lower dose of the drug. Many women do well on these medications on low doses. That is why I like to prescribe a low dose of Prozac. Prozac, or fluoxetine, comes in a tablet. It can be cut in half. Other drugs that come in a tablet are Paxil and Lexapro. Wellbutrin is also wonderful and may have the least amount of sexual side effects. It comes in a low-dose 75 mg capsule. Many of the drugs used for breast cancer are antiestrogens and cause a decrease in libido. The medication is designed to decrease the estrogen in your body which makes the vaginal mucosa (skin) thin and decreases the blood supply to the area. The following drugs and drug classes may cause a decrease in desire:

Antipsychotics	(Risperdal, Seroquel, Thorazine)
Barbiturates	(Nembutal, Phenobarbital, Seconal)
Benzodiazepines	(Xanax, Valiu, Klonopin)
Bipolar disorder	(Lithium)
SSRIs	(Prozac, Lexapro, Zoloft)
TCA	(Elavil, Tofranil, Sinequan)
Sedative, antidepressant	(Desyrel, Trazodone)
Venlafaxin	(Effexor)
Anti-lipid meds	(Crestor, Lipitor)
Beta-blockers	(metoprolol, labetolol)
Blood pressure meds	(Clonidine, Methyldopa)
Heart rhythm drug	(Digoxin)
Diuretic	(Spironolactone)
Anti-androgen	(Danazol)
GnRh agonists	(Lupron)

Oral contraceptive pills	(many brands)
H2 blockers	(Zantac, Pepcid)
Pro-motility agents	(Reglan)
Indomethacin	(Indocin)
Anti-fungal meds	(Ketoconazole)
Anti-seizure meds	(Dilantin)
Aromatase inhibitors	(Arimidex, Aromasin, Femara)
Chemotherapy agents	(Tamoxifen)

The following drugs or drug classes may affect the ability to have an orgasm: antipsychotics, barbiturates, benzodiazepines, lithium, SSRIs, tricyclic antidepressants, MAO inhibitors, trazadone, venlafaxine, digoxin, methyldopa, antiandrogens, amphetamines (Adipex, Vyvanse, Adderal), and narcotics (Percocet, Lortab, Vicodin, Norco).

Grief affects libido. Grief is a more common emotion as we age. As we get older we know of more people that have become sick, got cancer or terrible diseases, and died. There are events in life that are hard to overcome. Perhaps your children did not turn out as if you had hoped they would. Maybe you lost a long-time job that you loved. Maybe many family members and friends have died and you cannot get over the grief and loss. You see your physician to treat your grief and low libido and they put you on an antidepressant which may promply lower your libido and may make it impossible to have an orgasm. Sometimes you just can't win.

In women the desire to have intercourse is multifactorial. When you are overcome with grief about anything, pleasuring yourself seems out of the question. Many types of emotional turmoil may affect every part of a woman. I think that so many women are overwhelmed in their lives. I am not sure that it is any different from fifty years ago, but it seems like it is worse. We may have reached some equality in the workplace, but we did not give anything up. The feminist revolution in the sixties and seventies was positive for women; however, while they were screaming for equal pay for equal jobs, they should have been screaming for men to help with the household. I bet men were just happy as clams. "Sure let them work hard outside the house, pay them the same as men, just make sure you do the housework when you get home." And we were happy to do it. We were stupid. No wonder women are overwhelmed. We have all the housework, most of the care of the children, taking care of another adult (husband) so that they are happy, and we have jobs as well. Therefore, we clock out at work, get home, and clock back in to our second shift. Women make sure the dinner is done and put away, and they do the laundry and clean. They then fall in bed just in time for their husbands to give them a poke and say, "Hey, are you ready for some fun?" Are you out of your mind? Women are overworked, overwhelmed, and underappreciated. I do not think that you have to look too far to find out why they have no libido.

55

WOMEN WHO WANT SEX AND HAVE A PARTNER WHO WANTS SEX

For the most part this is the rarest of the five types of women. It is extremely rare after menopause. In fact I really only have seen a few in the last seven years that I have been concentrating on menopausal medicine. The one patient who comes to mind has become a good friend over the past twenty years. We have been through a lot together. She has confided in me, and I have confided in her. At one of her visits her husband called her while she was on the exam table. She asked if she could take the call. I overheard him say, "We should celebrate!" She smiled and replied, "Yes! Of course!" She hung up and apologized for taking the call. I asked what she was celebrating. She said, "We find something every day to celebrate by having intercourse! It is our excuse for having sex as much as possible." I said, "What are you celebrating today?" She said, "My new haircut." I told her to stay away from any symptomatic menopausal women in the waiting room with guns. She told me that she would.

MY ADVICE FOR WOMEN AND MEN

56
ADVICE FOR WOMEN

So, after all of this information, what is my advice for women? I frequently tell my patients the following. If we could go back in time for just a minute to an era when patients just did what their doctor ordered and did not question their recommendation, this is what I would say. For those of you who have built up a lifetime of resentment and anger toward your husband, you have to reconcile and forgive. It is hard to admit that pent-up anger over the years of your marriage can make you hate to have sex, but when I sit down and really listen to why women do not like to have sex, they mention how they have been treated. They feel useless and used. If there is no help around the house for years and it is "expected" of them to have sex before going to bed, it becomes just another chore. If there has been no attention given to her personal pleasure, then sex is a chore. Talk to your priest, pastor, minister, rabbi, counselor, or whomever you confide in and admit your anger that has built up for years. Get a plan to let go of the anger and resentment; you may be trying to "punish" him for whatever has happened in the past by withholding and "hating" to have sex.

If this is your situation, then accept that you are also hurting yourself by refusing to be honest and work on the relationship. Plan an evening that you and your husband can sit down and really talk. Do not get on the computer, the phone, or turn on the television. You need to start over and put the past behind you. Forgive him for what he has done to you, and he needs to forgive you for the things that have upset him during your marriage. You have to let every bad memory go away. It is hard to do; it may be the most difficult thing that you have ever done in your life. If you need to get counseling for this, then do it. I tell my patients all the time to go to a psychologist at least once a year. Tell this person all the things that piss you off, get everything off your chest, and know that it is confidential. It is so exhilarating to let all that weight off your shoulders and put it on someone who is not your best friend and will not judge you. You do not have to worry about seeing them somewhere socially and being worried that you should not have told them something. A best friend is great for this, but she will always remember what you said about your relationship or your husband. Most of the time, that is okay, but really getting it all out helps you have the catharsis that most of us need. The counselor will also help you find the underlying cause of your anger or fears, and help you deal with it. Your best friend can listen, but cannot always help you with solutions. Please let go of the anger that has been pent-up for years; it is hurting you as much as it is hurting him. Start right now working on the relationship with your husband.

On the other hand, if you are in a bad and dysfunctional relationship, and, if you cannot let go of the resentment and anger, then maybe it is time for you to leave. Many women who are married to alcoholics (and/or emotionally and verbally abusive men) live horrible lives. Their husbands are different people when they are drinking or abusive, and they behave differently in private than they do in public. They know the man that they married is in there somewhere, and there is always the hope that he will stop drinking or stop being degrading to them. Some women come in and wish that their husbands would hit them. I know that this may sound bizarre if you are not in one of these relationships, but the reason that they want to be hit is so that they have some proof of the abuse. Verbal and emotional abuse is hard to prove. No one knows what happens behind closed doors. These women tell me that they meet their husbands at the door with their favorite drink, because if they help them get drunk faster, the abuse will only last until they pass out. This is a horrible way to live, but these very strong, but very sad women, keep the family together for the children and/or because they feel that there is no way out. If you are that unhappy, it is time for you to make some changes that will make you happy, especially if the children are gone. Give yourself permission to be happy; you deserve it. If you are in a physically sexually abusive relationship or emotionally abused, get out as soon as possible. Please get help now.

If you want to help your marriage, put as much effort into your relationship as you do your e-mail and Facebook time. It really needs to be given more emphasis than you are giving. You can still devote your time and energy to the children, but carve out daily time for your intimate partner. Start now. You will be amazed at how one sentence about how much you admire him will build him up inside. Give him attention every day. Do not let him go out of the house without complimenting him in some way. You will be shocked at how quickly small comments will improve his attitude. Make sure that you tell him that you respect him (and what he does for the family) when appropriate.

er what men worry about that may affect their outward display of love for you. He may be out of shape, tired, or have a low testosterone level and does not want you to think of him as "less of a man." Perhaps he is depressed about something. Women are much better at saying, "I am depressed." Men may not want to admit that they are depressed for fear of not being "manly." Pressure, resentment, and anger from work or toward a coworker may be consuming his thoughts at home. He may not want to put these worries or perhaps financial worries on you. Be cognizant that prior to about age sixty, a man's self-worth is directly related to his net worth. Financial pressures and comparison of himself to his friends may be consuming.

From a sexual standpoint, it is difficult for a man to be rejected sexually, even if it is his wife. If you are continually saying "no" to his sexual advances, maybe he is becoming too scared to ask you. Think of it as a Pavlov's dog analogy. If the dog is yelled at each time it rolls over on his belly for a belly rub, he probably will stop rolling over. A man needs sexual release just as you need emotional release. When a man asks for sex and is rejected, it is embarrassing. Whether he admits it, most men have a fear that he will not be able to satisfy his partner. Do you give him signals while making love that what he is doing feels good? Do you ever tell him that what he is doing is perfect or not to stop because he is making you feel so good? Positive reinforcement is great for a man; how else will he know how he is doing? Men fear that they will lose their erection during intercourse and fear that they will not be able to ejaculate. This gets worse the older that they get. Erectile dysfunction drugs have helped significantly in this area. For many men, however, it is difficult for them to ask their physician for help. It is important never to ridicule your husband when it comes to making love and never compare him to other men. This works both ways of course. No one wants to think of your spouse comparing you to other lovers that they have had. Also, remember that talking about problems that you are having and nagging has no place in the bedroom. Nothing will turn a man off faster that nagging and criticism. We tend to get in habits of nagging, and when we have someone cornered, it is easy to take the opportunity to get things off your chest. Keep your bedroom a place to love and take care of each other. Sit at the kitchen table or a home office to have intense or potentially volatile conversations. The bedroom is not a place to discuss the fact that you make more money than he makes. It is not a place to brag or embellish on the fact that you are better at anything. Men need to feel that they are the king of the world in the bedroom; this is the one place to build him up and show him respect. If you do, the emotional love that you crave will be much more accessible. It does not work if you insist that you will only respect him after he shows his love to you. On the other hand, it does not work for him if he will only show you emotional love after you show him respect. Pay it forward. This always works better and is more satisfying. Do not assume that he knows how you feel about him. Tell him how much you love him, how good he looks, and how wonderful he makes you feel. If you had a particularly great lovemaking session, tell him, and when you have a great orgasm, say, "Thank you!" This will make him feel great. The longer that you are together, the less you remember to tell each other these things. Everybody needs reassurance about love. If you give the reassurance to him, he will probably give it back to you. Men get embarrassed about their lack of physical fitness and being overweight just like women. How he feels about himself may be affecting his affection for you. Men do not talk about this as openly as women do, but he may not like himself naked either and may be embarrassed to be affectionate. You have to build him up. If you are overweight, and you know it, and you hate how you look, then start right now on changing your eating behavior. It is harder to lose weight after menopause; something horrible and terrible happens to our metabolism. There are many fad diets out there, but the fact of the matter is, you have to decrease your intake and increase your exercise. I know that I sound mean, but there is no other way to do it. Weight watchers and walking are a good way to start. Meal plans such as Jenny Craig and Nutrisystem are great in that it teaches you portion control. If you watch the news, you know that obesity is a terrible problem in America. A big part of the problem is the large portions that we have become accustomed to with each meal. There are great apps that you can download to your phone to watch your calories. Try to keep your calories under 1200 kcal per day. It is very hard to do, but when you realize that you can eat lots of good stuff and not much of the bad stuff, you will change your behavior. When you hate how you look, you do not want to be sensual and you surely do not want to have intercourse. Men feel the same way. If your husband is overweight and not very sexual, he may just be embarrassed about the way he looks.

If you have tried and tried and cannot do it on your own, then consider surgery. Lap-band surgery and gastric bypass surgery have come a long way. There are minimally invasive surgeries (just an incision in your belly button) that can give you the help that you need. The risks of being overweight may exceed the risks of the surgery. Please consult your physician about this surgery. If the physician does not know enough about it, then do some research and find someone who does. Most of the larger hospitals have seminars put on by their bariatric centers to educate the public on their services. Some insurance companies are even covering laparoscopic bariatric (lap-band) surgery now. You do not know if you do not inquire. I have seen so many patient's lives turned around by lap-band surgery and gastric bypass surgery. They are usually surprised by my recommendation because they do not consider themselves overweight enough to consider surgery.

When you feel good about yourself, you will feel better about making love. I have women come in saying that both she and her husband are too large to have vaginal-penile intercourse. They do other things to feel good, such as oral stimulation or intercourse between her breasts or buttocks; but they are both humiliated. This is a good situation for both husband and wife to go on a portion control diet. I also have several couples that did gastric bypass surgery. One of them goes first and the other takes care of them postoperatively. Once that person has recovered, the other one gets their surgery. The bond that this creates is difficult to recreate. You both can support each other in so many ways. It can be done. I have seen it happen. Start today.

If you do not feel sexy, then do something to fix it. Give yourself a manicure and/or pedicure or, if you can afford it, go get one. Get a new and fashionable haircut, go out, and get some new clothes or lingerie. Men get aroused quickly when they think of sex and see something sexy. Having your husband look at you and think about sex makes any woman feel better about herself. Being sexy requires some self-confidence and self-esteem. What don't you like about yourself? You have to answer truthfully and work on fixing the problems.

When you are in the bedroom and making love, let go!! Modesty has absolutely no place in your bedroom. Be uninhibited!

Men are stimulated by sight. Let him see you get undressed, take a shower in front of him (or with him), put lotion on your whole body in front of him, and even put on a dab of lubricant or moisturizer into your vagina while he is watching! You will probably not get the chance to put on your nightclothes for a while. Act sexy even if you don't feel that way. Get the angel out of the bedroom and be a naughty girl! Undress him yourself and be the initiator for once (especially if you have turned him down the last couple of nights). Do a strip-tease act and don't let him touch you until you are through with removing your clothes. Be brave, do something crazy such as installing a strip pole in your bedroom while he is at work, and greet him with a negligee, candles, and a bottle of champagne! You can even take lessons on pole dancing, and it can really help you lose weight. Kill two birds with one stone! Again, let go in the bedroom! Be wild and crazy! Be self-confident enough to initiate sex. It is okay to act erotic, talk a little nasty, and chase him around the bed. Men are very visual and a change of pace will arouse him.

When you are done with having children, or around the age of forty, get a Mirena IUD. This is when the PMS and the abnormal bleeding begins. If you are among the 90 percent of women who hardly have a period, you will probably be as happy as I am. If you are not having periods, you tend not to have PMS. You are still going to go through puberty in reverse, and we can handle those symptoms when they arise. I can give you low-dose Xanax for anxiety, low-dose Ambien for sleep, and a low-dose antidepressant (Prozac, Effexor, Paxil, Wellbutrin, or Lexapro) for mood swings and the inevitable rage that accompanies the complete and total demise of your ovaries. If your symptoms become intolerable, and you, after knowing the risks of estrogen and progesterone (HRT), decide to take these drugs, you probably can wean off the other medications.

Start using a vaginal estrogen to protect your vagina from thinning around age fifty. Remember, we are in the Viagra age and you have to be able to do "it" for the next thirty to forty years. If you and your partner are not having intercourse at least once a week, then I think that you should use a vibrator to keep your vagina stretched out and use the vibration to help keep up the blood flow to the area. You should also use the vibrator to have a good, quick orgasm, which will improve your overall well-being, diffuse your rage, and is not messy.

Use an arousal oil prior to intercourse to get the blood flowing to your labia and clitoris (the erectile tissue) as it may help you have an orgasm. Tell your husband at some point in your marriage how to make you have an orgasm. Make him give you one first (if he can wait) so that you do not go to sleep pissed off and frustrated. If he just cannot make you have one, show him how to use the vibrator to do it. Ask him to give you one or more orgasms via clitoral stimulation after intercourse. If this is not an option in your marriage, then keep a vibrator in the bathroom. Finish yourself off quickly, tinkle (so that you do not get a bladder infection), and get back to bed, you have a big day tomorrow.

If you do start on systemic estrogen, you can keep your IUD in for the progesterone therapy and protect your uterus. I would recommend that you use a topical estrogen and, if you have a uterus, keep getting the Mirena IUD so that you do not have to take a pill. Try to wean down off your systemic estrogen dosage every six months to a year. If you eventually stop the systemic estrogen, no one will be happier than your gynecologist. It is a risky drug.

Protect your vagina as long as you live. Many older women find a partner later in life (and you can bet he will be on Viagra) and wish that they had kept it in shape.

Talk to your doctor about hyposexual desire disorder (HSDD). If you meet the criteria, you may want to consider the new drug Flibanserin or Addyi.

57
ADVICE FOR MEN

I think that this section is really just a compilation of the things that my patients tell me. First, I would like to start with things that you should not say. By the way, I did not make up this list; these are actual things that husbands have said to their wives. In fact, if you do say the following, you may never have sex with her again.

If you lose 20 pounds, I will pay for you to have a face-lift.

I wish that you looked more like _____ .

I wish that you weren't so fat.

I wish that you would "put out" just a little bit.

You look like your mother.

That _____ (nightgown, dress, bathing suit, and outfit) looks matronly.

Do not blow dry your balls and tell her that you are heating up her dinner.

When men accompany their wives into my exam room and want to talk about how "I" (the doctor) can improve her libido, I love to give them several pointers. Women need to feel loved and appreciated. The minimum that you should think about doing is the following:

In January, go to the grocery store and buy a small bouquet of discounted flowers from the water bucket near the checkout line. Bring them home and give them to your wife and say, "I just wanted you to know that I was thinking about you on the way home." Do not get any food or milk, just go to get the flowers.

In April send a card in the mail (using a postage stamp) to your wife saying that you love and appreciate everything that she does for you and that you want her to know that you love her very much.

In July stop and get the bouquet of flowers again.

In October, send a card again in the mail for no reason that says, "I love you."

When you want to have sex, she may not be in the mood, but she is going to think to herself, "He did send me that card a few months ago." Alternatively, "Gosh, he did bring those flowers home that day." I have said this so many times in the office with a woman nodding her head up and down, telling him to listen to me, and they come back and say, "He still didn't do it even after you told him to."

Women are begging for affection and love. They are so hungry for romance.

They want you to tell them that they are beautiful, even when they know that they are not. Women want you to tell them that they are sexy and that they turn you on. Do not assume that they know how you feel. On the inside, they are twenty-year-old coeds who are excited to be with you. Keep that excitement up. Do whatever you can to re-spark the romance. Why do you think the Harlequin Romances of many years ago were so popular? It is because we imagined ourselves in the heroine's place. We want to be swept off our feet in love every day, or at least once a month. Just as you may think about having sex every day, we think about romance every day.

I have read multiple articles and books on this subject to prepare for writing this book. All of them say that getting a new partner usually fixes a woman's problems with decreased desire; it is the excitement and the romance to which she is responding. However, she doesn't want a new partner. She wants you to be romantic again. She wants her husband to be her knight in shining armor! Come home a couple times a month and help do some household chores or start dinner; women do it every day. Small gestures of help will go a long way. Not many women come home from work to find the laundry done, the rugs vacuumed, and dinner ready. Most of them cannot imagine having this happen. (This could get you laid on the living room floor!)

I can remember visiting my brother and sister-in-law several years ago. We were sitting at the kitchen table with my late husband, his brother and his wife, their daughter and son-in-law, and their new baby. We were all talking and catching up on our lives when the baby started to get fussy. Their daughter said to everyone, "It is time to give him his bath and get him ready for bed. Their son-in-law got up, got the baby out of the high chair, and picked up the diaper bag. He started to go out of the room, and my husband and his brother said in unison, "Where the hell are you going?" The three women looked at each other in disbelief, and my sister-in-law said, "Unbelievably, he is going to help her!" They looked back at her and said, "Why?"

My patients who talk to me about these things are tired and feel unappreciated. You may think that it is too late to change things. It isn't too late. If it were too late, they would not be in my office talking about it. They are craving attention and romance. Give it to them. Show her how you appreciate her. Tell her how much you appreciate her. What person in the world, man or woman, doesn't feel good when someone says, "I appreciate what you do for me." It is the greatest feeling in the world. Give them something to talk about to their girlfriends. No woman in the world would love it more than to tell her friends that they think that you have gone crazy because all of a sudden you have become profoundly romantic.

You could see some jealous women! Be romantic in front of her friends and mean it. If you are in a restaurant and an old familiar song comes on, dance with her. Every woman in the restaurant will want to be in her shoes; they will all be jealous. Make her feel sexy and build up her self-esteem (a feeling of respect for yourself and your abilities) and self-confidence (confidence in oneself and in one's abilities). This may be one of the most difficult parts of the chapter. It is difficult to raise another person's self-confidence and self-esteem. We teach our daughters to be demure, modest, and maintain their dignity when they are dating; but we do not tell them that once they are married, they should be an animal in the bedroom. We drill into their heads that they need to maintain their self-respect and not act whorish. However, that is really what their husbands want! They want their wives to be an angel in public and an absolute devil in the bedroom. If you understand what women feel is expected of them, it is no wonder that they do not let go while having sex. Her only instruction in the art of making love may only be you and perhaps several inexperienced young men prior to your marriage. There has to be communication and a willingness to experiment with new things. Talk to her and tell her what you like; this is easier said than done.

The first thing to do is to make her feel like she is the best person in the world to you. Let her know that she is pretty, funny, sexy, or whatever she is to you. Build her up; we always assume that our partner knows how we feel about them. They don't. Let her hear it from you, often. Don't be selfish while making love; tell her and show her that you are more interested in her pleasure. Help her feel comfortable being naked. All women look in the mirror naked and can give a list of all the things that are wrong, ugly, or misshapen. Tell her how beautiful she is naked and how much you love to look at her naked. Once she is comfortable with herself and is not embarrassed, help her with her self-confidence. When she does something to you that makes you feel good, tell her! Say thank you and mean it. Tell her that you now want to make her feel just as good.

Never forget about the clitoris! It is unforgivable for a man to be ilcliterite! Talk to her about how you can move during intercourse to stimulate the clitoris. Experiment with different angles to try to get this to happen. If it doesn't happen, consider finding a small vibrator that she can hold in place to get the clitoral stimulation. Encourage her to move in ways to get the clitoral stimulation and be happy for her if she finds out how to do it. Have fun finding the sweet spot and laugh with each other!

Lubrication is a necessity. Let's think of a vagina as a car engine. Oil lubrication of your car engine is used to reduce friction on the metal parts by placing a film between those parts. The lubrication system in the car has to lubricate the parts continuously. Eventually the oil becomes thick and non-viscous; therefore, we have to change the oil so that the metal parts are not destroyed. If you fail to change the oil and keep up adequate levels for the engine to function, you will destroy the engine. The viscosity of the oil must be the correct mixture for that particular engine, for example 10W30, and the oil suitable for the severity of the operating conditions. If the oil is too thick, it will not flow through the engine parts fast enough to dissipate heat. The lubrication system is fed by the oil sump that forms the lower enclosure of the engine. Oil is taken from the sump by a pump, usually of the gear type, and is passed through a filter and delivered under pressure to a system of passages or channels drilled through the engine. Filtered oil is supplied under pressure to crankshaft and camshaft main bearings. Oil that is leaking from the crankshaft bearings is sprayed on the cylinder walls, cams, and up into the pistons to lubricate the piston pins. A spring-loaded pressure-relief valve maintains the pressure at the proper level. Guys, our oil sump is broken because the lower enclosure of our engine is not getting enough blood supply. Our pump, filter, crankshaft, camshaft, and pressure system needs to be replaced, but there are no spare parts to replace this anywhere in the world. Therefore, you have to keep this classic engine running with appropriate and great lubricants.

There are water-based and silicone lubricants that are specifically made for this purpose. Vaseline has too high a viscosity for most women, and water has too low a viscosity. Sometimes we need flavored or warming lubricants just because we want them that day. Our vaginas are a beautiful, rare, and complicated classic machine. Remember that so many things are going through our brains when you want to make love. We are tired and feel that the house has to be perfect. Help her get that done. We have anger, bitterness, and resentment towards others or you that may affect how we respond. Help her get through this and resolve it. Women also have fear of rejection in the bedroom. We are so self-critical it is very hard to let go completely; help her to feel beautiful and sexy.

I found some rules on the internet, which may let you understand our feelings about sex a little better.

These are the "golf rules of the bedroom."

1. Each player shall furnish his own equipment.

2. Play on a course must be approved by the owner of the hole.

3. Unlike outdoor golf, the object is to get the club in the hole and keep the balls out.

4. For most effective play, the club requires a firm shaft. Course owners may check shaft stiffness before play begins.

5. Course owners reserve the right to restrict club length to avoid damage to the hole.

6. The object of the game is to take as many strokes as necessary until the course owner is satisfied that play is completed. Failure to do so may result in being denied permission to play the course again.

7. It is considered bad form to begin playing the hole immediately upon arrival at the course. The experienced player will normally take time to admire the entire course with special attention to well-formed bunkers.

8. Players are cautioned not to mention other courses they have played or are currently playing to the owner of the current course. Upset course owners have been known to damage players' equipment.

9. Players are encouraged to bring proper rain gear for protection.

10. Players should ensure themselves that their match has been properly scheduled, particularly when a new course is being played for the first time. Previous players have been known to become irate if they discover someone else playing on what they considered their private course.

11. Players should not assume a course is in shape for play at all times. Some players may be embarrassed if they find the course to be temporarily under repair. Players are advised to be extremely tactful in this situation, while more advanced players will find alternative means of play.

12. The course owner is responsible for manicuring and pruning any bush around the hole to allow for improved viewing of, alignment with, and approach to the hole.

13. Players must obtain the course owner's permission before attempting to play the back nine.

14. Slow play is encouraged, but players should be prepared for quicker play, at least temporarily, at the course owner's request.

15. Time permitting, it is considered outstanding performance to play the same hole several times in one match.

I wish that I knew who wrote this, because it is perfect.

I really hate to say this, but it may help tremendously to take a shower and wash your "parts" well with soap. I know that this works both ways, but think of how we see men behave all day. When women greet each other, they may hug or even kiss each other's cheeks to say hello. However, we watch you greeting friends, acquaintances, business partners, new people, and just about everybody with a handshake. After twenty or more handshakes, you go to the bathroom, hold your penis in your hands, and then go wash your hands. Everyone's germs that you shook hands with are now on your penis. Then you come home and want to put it in our vaginas or mouths. It is not a pleasant thought.

Make a habit of washing your hands *before and after* you go to the bathroom, and make a point of taking a shower prior to getting in bed, especially if you want any oral favors. No one wants all the germs from everybody you met and shook hands with today in our vaginas or in our mouths. Sorry guys, but why do you think that women do not like to do this? How would you feel if your wife shook hands with twenty people, then came up, and asked you to lick the palm of her hand? Not so nice. Besides the germs, many women just feel that giving a blowjob is humiliating. They are not going to do it whether you wash it or not. That I cannot fix. That is why there is chocolate and vanilla. Different people like to do different things. There are lubricants and products that you can use on your penis to make it more "palatable." Flavored lubricants come in hot buttered rum and cosmopolitan flavors. (What woman doesn't want a cosmo?) There are whiskey-flavored condoms, or you could try some whipped cream or chocolate. All women feel better when we have had some chocolate. You never know. It could work. Shave your face before going to bed (especially if you want to give any oral favors). Some women may like the scratchiness, but I bet most of us would like you to kiss us all over and rub your faces on our faces and places with soft skin. Some tissues are very sensitive.

If you cannot maintain an erection, then do other things. First, don't wait five years before you try an erectile-dysfunction drug. Ask your doctor for help as soon as you have some erectile dysfunction. If you wait years and your wife has not had anything stretching out the vagina, it is going to get smaller. When you do get the nerve up to get some, she will not be able to do it anymore.

If these products don't work, remember, it is not all about the vaginal penetration; it is about the romance. Use a vibrator in place of your penis and ask her how to use it right. Don't feel like you are a failure because you are not the one in the vagina. She will respect you more because you can admit the obvious instead of ignoring the obvious. She will be in heaven and actually respect you more if you are confident enough in yourself to admit that it doesn't work the way it used to when you were younger. Just because your parts don't work well doesn't mean that our parts don't work well. You like to have an orgasm, and we do too. The worst thing that you can do is assume that just because you can't do it, then we don't want it. You would hate it if your wife said, "I'm not doing any more hand jobs or having oral sex on you because I can't have an orgasm anymore. Unfortunately this is how many of my patients live. So many women come into the office and say that their husbands cannot maintain an erection, so they have to do it for them by hand or with their mouths. Because there is no reciprocity, they feel resentful and used; it becomes like a chore to help you have an orgasm. When you are finished, consider saying, "Now it's your turn."

Remember that in order for a woman to have an orgasm, the clitoris must be stimulated. For most women this is the only way that she can have an orgasm. The clitoris is analogous to the penis in men; can you imagine having sex and not having your penis touched at all? Many women live this way. If your penis were never touched, you would become frustrated and not look forward to having sex. If you do not touch the clitoris, this is how women feel. It takes a long time for a woman to have the first orgasm, but once she does, the next ones will be quicker and probably more intense. I know that it is not fair that she can have pretty much as many orgasms in one sexual encounter that she can stand, but you should take advantage of this fact. It is unconscionable for a man to be ilcliterate.

We really need lots and lots of foreplay; it is essential. Think of it as football. It is not just the kickoff for you, is it? If the game starts at 3:30 P.M., you may start preparing for the game at 12:00 noon. The cooler needs to be filled with beer and iced down. You must give this several hours to be at the right temperature. You have to call your favorite friends to come over, and you must prepare the chips and dip. The hamburgers have to be ready to put on the grill at half-time so that you can be finished eating before the second half starts. The grill has to be checked to see if it is working properly and you need to make sure that you have plenty of propane. Once this is all in order, you can relax a little bit. You will not completely relax until all of the men are settled with beer in hand and sitting in front of the television just in time for the pregame show. Women learn early that the pregame show is an integral part of the football game. Foreplay for us is an integral part of the sexual game; it is our preparation and pregame show. It is our lead-up to the game. Think of the romancing as our preparation for the game and clitoral stimulation as the pregame show. Give her some warning that you want to make love to her. Let the "buildup" build up. She needs to feel ready. Let her anticipate what is coming. Tell her that she is beautiful; whisper in her ear and tickle her neck with your breath. Touch her gently, all over. Don't just dive to the prize. Some women can have an orgasm just by fondling her breasts and stimulating her nipples. Work up to touching her vulva and clitoris. The excitement of knowing what is coming but not knowing when it is coming is stimulating.

Remember, the longer you spend on the romantic part of making love, the more that we will love to make love. Once you have built up the excitement, you can sit down for the pregame show. If you help her have an orgasm first, she is going to relax and really enjoy what is coming next. Ask her what to do to her clitoris in order to make her have an orgasm. If she is too embarrassed to tell you what to do, then do things that you think she would like and listen to the signals. My suggestion is to take your middle finger or index finger on your dominant hand, keep place it on one side of her clitoris, and move your hand up and down y⁻ e plenty of lubricant when you do this; it hurts if everything is dry and rubbing. Do not push down hard as the tissue on the clitoris is very sensitive. Move your hand fast up and down without hooking your finger under the clitoris. If she is moaning in pleasure, keep it up; if she is not, try something else. Put your finger on the other side of the clitoris. Maybe try putting a finger on each side at the same time. She may like you to go side to side instead of up and down. Go fast, not hard. If this doesn't work, see how a vibrator works on her. I call them intimacy aids for a reason. They will help speed up the process to be intimate with you. Get a book and read about it. Watch a YouTube video on how to give a woman an orgasm. Learn. I can't say it enough. Once she has had an orgasm, she is ready for the game. No matter how much you may worry about it, a vibrator or manual clitoral stimulation will not take the place of you being inside her vagina. Women need the closeness of holding their husbands while they are inside them. It is the ultimate statement to her that you love her. It should be done with compassion and the promise of sexual satisfaction for both of you.

It's all about the romance! Romance. Romance. Romance. Intimacy, affection, love, and romance will get you anywhere you want to go. I can't say it enough! Get an old romance novel and read some of it. Find out what we like to read about and try to do something similar. Turn off the television while having dinner and actually talk to her. With twenty-four-hour news stations, DVRs and TiVo, there is no reason to watch the news after someone has made you dinner. Please, sit down and talk.

Suggest lighting some candles and having a glass of wine with dinner while you talk.

Take a walk around the block and hold hands.

Take a walk and hold hands on the beach.

Take a walk in the rain.

Go to the beach at night with a blanket, look at the stars, listen to the surf, and tell her how much you love her.

Make love to her in the dunes on the beach.

Bring a bottle of champagne to the beach at night and just talk.

Go to the beach at night with a CD player and a blanket. Play some beach music and shag dance. (This will make a 'Southern Girl' get naked quickly.)

Make a picnic dinner with wine, eat it in the sand dunes at night under the moonlight, and listen to the surf.

Kiss her lying down in the surf like Cary Grant.

Drive to the beach, sit in a chair next to each other, and hold her hand.

On a cold night, make hot chocolate; sit in front of a fire with a blanket over both of you, and cuddle.

Make a picnic lunch (go out and buy the picnic basket and the blanket) and pick her up from work and surprise her. If you do this in front of her co-workers, you could get laid in public on the blanket.

Take her to the mall for a shopping spree and then dinner.

Take her to New York City and let her shop on 5th Avenue.

Take her to a Broadway show in New York.

Go to a lake or river and row her in a small boat.

Learn how to play a new sport together (golf, racquetball, or tennis).

Train for a 5K together.

Build a sand castle together.

Take her to a butterfly garden or a butterfly house.

Go on a hike together and pack a picnic lunch.

Pack a picnic lunch and take a blanket to her office; have a picnic on the floor in her office if she can't leave.

Leave love notes around the house.

Read a romantic book to her; one chapter a night.

Read an erotic book together.

Put a blindfold on her and surprise her by driving her to a place that is special to both of you.

Get side-by-side pedicures (women love men to have nice feet and nails).

Go horseback riding.

Make her breakfast in bed on the weekend.

Bring her coffee and have it next to the bed when she wakes up.

When she wakes up, have a robe and slippers ready.

Get a hammock and relax together.

Get in a hot tub naked and drink champagne.

If you have a pool, go skinny-dipping.

Write a song about your love and sing it to her.

Take her to New York City and sing to her on the top of the Empire State Building.

Rent a log cabin in the mountains for a weekend.

Pick blackberries on a deserted road.

Take her for a snowmobile ride.

Make snow angels side by side.

Take a horse-drawn carriage ride.

Rent a limousine and take her out for a special evening.

Take her to the place where you were engaged and ask her to marry you all over again.

Take her to the place that you had your first date.

Pick wildflowers, put them in a vase, and give them to her.

Surprise her with a trip to a country that she has always wanted to visit.

Karaoke her while at a karaoke bar with your wedding song. (This could get you laid in the bar.)

Praise her in front of your friends and mean it.

Praise her in front of her friends and mean it.

Write letters to her explaining in your own words what makes you more in love with her now than when you were married.

Take her to a museum and hire a private tour guide to explain the art. Bring a bottle of champagne and pretty glasses to enjoy during the tour.
Surprise her with chocolate covered strawberries and champagne in your bed room. Light some candles to set the mood.

Do a strip tease dance in the bedroom.

Romance. Romance. Romance.

Refer to sex as "making love." It just makes us feel better about ourselves, our relationship, and especially about you.

Get the idea of making love on our "to do list" at the beginning of the day… not at the end of the day when we are crawling in bed and falling asleep before our halos hit the pillow.

Good luck!

BIBLIOGRAPHY

CHAPTER 8 (EXPERIENCES OF A LIFETIME)
Anna's Mother. Unsolicited opinions. 1977–present.

Hardy, E., L. Bahamondes, M. J. Osis, R. G. Costa, and A. Faundes. "Risk Factors for Tubal Sterilization Regret, Detectable Before Surgery." *Contraception*, vol. 54, issue 3 (September 1996), 159–62.

Peterson, Herbert B., Zhisen Xis, Joyce M. Hughes, Lynne S. Wilcox, Lisa Ratliff Tylor and For the U.S. Collaborative Review of Sterilization Working Group. "The Risk of Pregnancy After Tubal Sterilization: Findings From the U.S. Collaborative Review of Sterilization." *American Journal of Obstetrics and Gynecology*, vol. 174, issue 4 (April 1996), 1161–70.

CHAPTER 19 (THE SPECULUM)
Baskett, Thomas F. *On the Shoulders of Giants: Eponyms and Names in Obstetrics and Gynaecology*. (London: RCOG Press, 1996). 23–24, 209–210.

Cianfrani, Theodore. *A Short History of Obstetrics and Gynecology*. (Springfield, Ill.: Charles C. Thomas, Publisher, Bannerstone House, 1960), 331–38.

Döderlein, Günter. *Antique Medical Instruments*. (Tuttlingen, Germany: Aesculap-Werke AG, n.d.), p. 14.

CHAPTER 24 (THE VULVA)
"Managing Common Vulvar Skin Conditions," *Harvard Women's Health Watch*, vol. 16, no. 3 (November 2008), 3–5.

CHAPTER 27 (PERIMENOPAUSE)
Casper, Robert F., Robert L. Barbieri, William F. Crowley, and Kathryn A. Martin. "Clinical Manifestations and Diagnosis of Menopause." (Wolters Kluwer, UpToDate, 2014).

CHAPTER 29 (TREATING THE BLEEDING)
Sharp, Walter T., Tommaso Falcone, and Sandy J. Falk. "An Overview of Endometrial Ablation." (Wolters Kluwer, UpToDate, 2014).

Chapter 30 (Progesterone IUDS)
Caursi, Daniela A., Alisa B. Goldverg, Mimi Zieman, and Vanessa A. Barss. "Insertion and Removal of an Intrauterine Contraceptive Device." (Wolters Kluwer, UpToDate, 2014).

Dean, Gillian, Alisa B. Goldberg, Mimi Zieman, and Vanessa A. Barss. "Management of Problems Related to Intrauterine Contraception." (Wolters Kluwer, UpToDate, 2014).

————. "Overview if Intrauterine Contraception." (Wolters Kluwer, UpToDate, 2014).

Chapter 31 (Menopause)
Casper, Robert F., Robert L. Barbieri, William F. Crowley, and Kathryn A. Martin. "Clinical Manifestations and Diagnosis of Menopause." (Wolters Kluwer, UpToDate, 2014).

Chapter 32 (Memory Loss)
Shadlen, Marie-Florence, Eric B. Larson. Steven T. DeKosky, Kenneth E. Schmader, and April F. Eichler. "Evaluation of Cognitive Impairment and Dementia." (Wolters Kluwer, UpToDate, 2014.

Chapter 34 (Protect Your Vagina)
Bachmann, Gloria, Richard J. Santen, Robert L. Barbeiri, and Sandy J. Falk. "Clinical Manifestations and Diagnosis of Vaginal Atrophy." (Wolters Kluwer, UpToDate, 2013).

————. "Treatment of Vaginal Atrophy." (Wolters Kluwer, UpToDate, 2013). Casper, Robert F. "Clinical Manifestations and Diagnosis of Menopause." (Wolters Kluwer, UpToDate, 2014).

Pritchard, Kathleen I., Daniel Hayes, and Don S. Dizon. "Adjuvant Endocrine Therapy for Non-metastatic Hormone Receptor-positive Breast Cancer." (Wolters Kluwer, UpToDate, 2014).

CHAPTER 36 (SYSTEMIC ESTROGEN)
Writing Group for the Women's Health Initiative Investigators. "Risks and Benefits of Estrogen Plus Progestin in Healthy Postmenopausal Women: Principal Results from the Women's Health Initiative Randomized Controlled Trial." *Journal of the American Medical Association (JAMA)*, vol. 288, no. 3 (July 17, 2002), 321–33. www.health.harvard.edu/newsweek/Postmenopausal_hormones_Hormone_therapy.htm

CHAPTER 38 (HOW DOES YOUR OB/GYN REALLY FEEL ABOUT ESTROGEN?)
Bachmann, Gloria, Richard J. Santen, Robert L. Barbeiri, and Sandy J. Falk. "Clinical Manifestations and Diagnosis of Vaginal Atrophy." (Wolters Kluwer, UpToDate, 2013).

———. "Treatment of Vaginal Atrophy." (Wolters Kluwer, UpToDate, 2013).

Martin, Kathryn A., and Robert A. Barbieri. "Preparations for Postmenopausal Hormone Therapy." (Wolters Kluer, UpToDate, 2014).
Osphena Drug Pamphlet 2013

Writing Group for the Women's Health Initiative Investigators. "Risks and Benefits of Estrogen Plus Progestin in Healthy Postmenopausal Women: Principal Results from the Women's Health Initiative Randomized Controlled Trial." *Journal of the American Medical Association (JAMA)*, vol. 288, no. 3 (July 17, 2002), pp. 321–33.

CHAPTER 40 (HERBAL ALTERNATIVES)
Bachmann, Gloria, Richard J. Santen, Robert L. Barbeiri, and Sandy J. Falk. "Treatment of Vaginal Atrophy." (Wolters Kluwer, UpToDate, 2013).

Casper, Robert F., Richard J. Santen, Robert L. Barbieri, and William F. Crowley, and Kathryn A. Martin. "Menopausal Hot Flashes." (Wolters Kluwer, UpToDate, 2014).

Martin, Kathryn A., Robert L. Barbieri, Peter J. Synder, and William F. Crowley. "Preparations for Postmenopausal Hormone Therapy." (Wolters Kluwer, UpTo Date, 2014).

Reed, Susan D., and N. D. Guiltinian. "Herbal Altrenatives for Menopausal Symptoms." *Contemporary OB/GYN.* (November 2010), 38–46.

Santen, Richard J., Peter J. Synder, William F. Crowley, and Kathryn A. Martin. "Patient Information: Non-hormonal Treatments for Menopausal Symptoms (Beyond the Basics)." (Wolters Kluwer, UpToDate, 2014).

www.health.harvard.edu/newsweek/what-are-bioidentical-hormones.htm

CHAPTER 42 (PROGESTERONES)
DuaVee package insert

Martin, Kathryn A., Robert L. Barbieri, Peter J. Snyder, and William F. Crowley. "Preparations for Postmenopausal Hormone Therapy." (Wolters Kluwer, UpToDate, 2014).

CHAPTER 43 ((MALE HORMONES)
Shifren, Jan L., Robert L. Barbieri, William F. Crowley, and Sandy J. Falk. "Sexual Dysfunction in Women: Epidemiology, Risk Factors, and Evaluation." (Wolters Kluwer, UpToDate, 2013).

————. "Sexual Dysfunction in Women: Management." (Wolters Kluwer, UpToDate, 2014).

Udoff, Laurence C., Robert L. Barbeiri, William F. Crowley, and Kathryn A. Martin. "Androgen Production and Therapy in Women." (Wolters Kluwer, UpToDate, 2013).

CHAPTER 45 (ANGER AND SLEEP MANAGEMENT)
Bradford, Andrea. Robert Segraves, and Richard Hermann. "Female Orgasmic Disorder: Epidemiology, Pathogenesis, Clinical Manifestations, Course, Assessment, and Diagnosis." (Wolters Kluwer, UpToDate, 2014).

Hirsch, Michael, Robert J. Birnbaum, Peter P. Roy-Byrne, and David Solomon. "Sexual Dysfunction Associated with Selective Serotonin Re-uptake Inhibitor (SSRI) Antidepressants: Management." (Wolters Kluwer, UpToDate, 2014).

CHAPTER 46 (THE ORGASM)
http://robtshepoherd.tripod.com/marie-robinson.html

Robinson, Marie N. *The Power of Sexual Surrender* (New York: New American Library, 1958).

CHAPTER 54 (WOMEN WHO DON'T WANT SEX AND WHO ARE WITH MEN WHO DO)
Buster, John E. "Sex and the 50-something Woman: Strategies for Restoring Satisfaction," *Contemporary OB/GYN* (August 2012), pp. 32–39.

Iverson, Robert E., Jr., Alan H. DeCherney, Robert L. Barbieri, and Sandy J. Falk. "Clinical Manifestations and Diagnosis of Congenital Anomalies of the Uterus." (Wolters Kluwer, UpToDate, 2014).

Kingsberg, Sheryl A. , et al. "Female Sexual Disorders: Enhancing Communication Skills." MPR Obstetricians and Gynecologist edition. CME Activity, November 2010.

Laufer, Marc R., Robert L. Barbieri, and Sandy J. Falk, "Diagnosis and Management of Congenital Anomalies of the Vagina." (Wolters Kluwer, UpToDate, 2014).

ABOUT THE AUTHOR

PAMELA DEE GAUDRY, MD, FACOG, NCMP, graduated summa cum laude from the University of Georgia in 1985. She received her medical degree from the Medical College of Georgia in 1989 and completed her internship and residency there in 1993. Dr. Gaudry received many honors while in residency, including "Intern of the Year" and "Junior Resident of the Year." During her senior year she was awarded "Senior Resident of the Year," won the resident thesis award, and served as chief administrative resident.

Dr. Gaudry has been on the faculty of Memorial University Medical Center in Savannah, Georgia, since completing her residency in 1993 and currently holds the title of Assistant Professor of Obstetrics and Gynecology for Mercer University School of Medicine (MUSM).

Dr. Gaudry has been active in the Georgia OB/GYN Society since 1993, has served on the Board of Directors since 1996, and was president of the Society in 2007, representing over 1,400 OB/GYN physicians. She has been a delegate to the Medical Association of Georgia's House of Delegates for over a decade.

Dr. Gaudry has been a member of the Georgia Medical Society and served as president of this Society representing over 600 physicians in the Chatham, Effingham, and Bryan counties of Georgia.

Dr. Gaudry served as the First and Second Vice President of the Medical Association of Georgia. She was a member of the inaugural class of the Georgia Physician Leadership Academy in 2007. She served as Vice Chair and Chair of the Georgia Section of the American College of Obstetricians and Gynecologists for a total of six years.

Dr. Gaudry is a NAMS-certified menopause practitioner and is a Florida State Certified Sex Therapist. She is a board-certified Fellow of the American College of Obstetricians and Gynecologists, as well as a member of the North American Menopause Society, the Sexual Medicine Society of North America, and the International Society of the Study of Women's Sexual Health. She loves her patients, her "honeybears" as she calls them, with all of her heart and rarely does anyone get out of her office without a bear hug. Affectionately known to her patients as "Dr. Pam," she resides in Savannah, Georgia, where she devotes her practice to the care of menopausal women. She is on a mission to save not only long-term marriages, but the intimacy and romance that is sometimes lost over time.

Special Acknowledgment by Reverent June Juliet Gatlin

Beloved Dr. Pam,

Thank You for writing, sharing Your Love, Sweat and Tears with Us. It is A Dynamic and Divinely Inspiring Affirmation, A full service book Honoring The Female Human—And Her Body Temple.

We appreciate the manner in which you give care-filled attention to the unique connectivity of Woman's whole Being, Her PhysicalMentalEmotional Body whilst defining fluctuating moments so searing and complex She, oftentimes, does not comprehend what is happening.

You are disseminating definitive, insightful, and self-edifying information pertaining to the intimate intricacies of Woman's sacred spaces; information relevant regarding Her *most mysterious, complex and scariest occurrence: Menopause.*

Oh, yes, it be about The Blood, Dear Sisters, the coming, going and ceasing of The Blood and those powerful change of life disturbances can be quite threatening. Countless Bodies have a hell of a time adjusting to *The Hot Flushes.*

You certainly have Your loving way and it's good.

Every Body should have some Love Sweat and Tears moments especially the manner in which you fearlessly stomp all over old ways and myths, how to, not to, do not do, the why didn't I and why shouldn't we or can we.

You generously give the down to earth no holds barred grittiness of Sex, recommending and encouraging Women and Men to acknowledge their Oneness, telling it's okay to communicate about those hidden places usually experienced only when ready to come together sexually. You also define the hot and heavy, sweaty moments as well as those listless times when She doesn't feel like "doing it", not up to even when He would like to get up and go down. Love, Sweat and Tears tells about the soreness, the sour, salty and the spicy and it can definitely be about The Plush Lush Loving Life too.

You want Loving Humans to know there is not a right or wrong way involving Vagina and Penis; there is only Their way.

Thank You for sharing a delicate definitive about Women, Our Bodies. And Our Loving Men.

Dr. Pam, You are The Best.

Thank You for helping, assisting, showing and telling about The Fullness of Woman's Journey, presenting an invitation for dialogue and discussion about Life's Nectar: The Blood.

You're inviting Man and Woman to unite within Mind Body and Soul to Recognize, Appreciate, Respect and Celebrate Menopause being A Spiritual Life Transformation Journey.

It's perfectly alright, good and a blessing to learn and know about Woman's special needs and precious priorities. And, if need be, folk may create discussion Groups because, actually, Women and Men require Help when Menopause arrives.

You have shown Dedication, Determination and Discipline while unfolding Your Brilliant work, lumps, bumps, scars, The whole Spiritual Adventure including Your God Wink. You are She who truly recognized, trusted and adhered to Your Spiritual Calling. Love Sweat and Tears compliments The gentleness of A Woman Doctor's Celebration of Life. Your words are likened to a Moving Picture.

Love, Sweat and Tears is a wonder filled Testimony to Life and All Its Radiant and Remarkable Majesty. Your Loving Life's Work is Appreciated.
Oh, and Menopause is not a joke (wink).

Loving You Always,

Reverent June Juliet Gatlin
Spiritual Advisor and Author